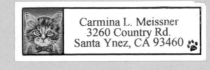

Carmina L. Meissner
3260 Country Rd.
Santa Ynez, CA 93460

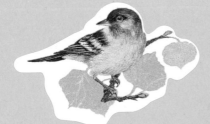

P9-CJC-556

THE
DANIEL
PLAN

COOKBOOK

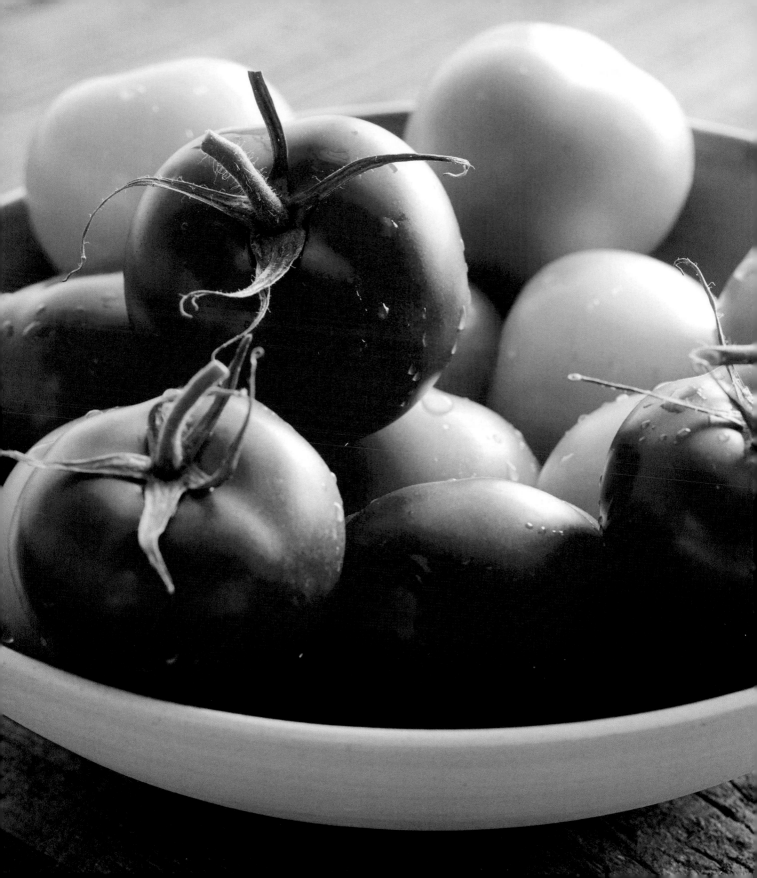

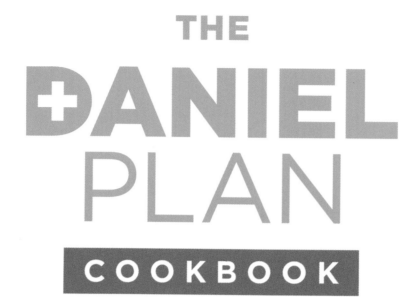

THE DANIEL PLAN COOKBOOK

HEALTHY EATING *for* LIFE

RICK WARREN D.MIN.
DANIEL AMEN M.D.
MARK HYMAN M.D.

featuring The Daniel Plan Signature Chefs,
SALLY CAMERON, JENNY ROSS, AND ROBERT STURM

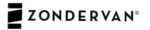

ZONDERVAN®

ZONDERVAN

The Daniel Plan Cookbook
Copyright © 2014 by The Daniel Plan

This title is also available as a Zondervan ebook.
Visit www.zondervan.com/ebooks.

Requests for information should be addressed to:

Zondervan, Grand Rapids, Michigan 49530

Library of Congress Cataloging-in-Publication Data

Warren, Rick.
    The Daniel Plan Cookbook: Healthy Eating for Life / Rick
Warren, D.Min., Daniel Amen, M.D., Mark Hyman, M.D. ; with
The Daniel Plan Signature Chefs, Sally Cameron, Jenny Ross,
and Robert Sturm.
       pages cm
    Includes index.
    ISBN 978-0-310-34426-1 (hardcover)
    1. Natural foods—Health aspects. 2. Natural foods—
Recipes. 3. Nutrition—Religious aspects—Christianity.
I. Amen, Daniel. II. Hyman, Mark. III. Title.
RM237.55.W36 2013
641.5'637—dc23   2013041228

All Scripture quotations, unless otherwise indicated, are taken
from The Holy Bible, New International Version®, NIV®. Copyright
© 1973, 1978, 1984, 2011 by Biblica, Inc.® Used by permission of
Zondervan. All rights reserved worldwide.

A medical disclaimer appears on page iv, which hereby becomes
part of this copyright page. Any Internet addresses (websites,
blogs, etc.) and telephone numbers printed in this book are
offered as a resource. They are not intended in any way to be
or imply an endorsement by Zondervan, nor does Zondervan
vouch for the content of these sites and numbers for the life of
this book.

Cover design: Curt Diepenhorst
Cover photo: Kent Cameron
Cover food styling: Sally Cameron
Interior photos: Photography and Styling by Matt Armendariz
   and Adam Pearson, unless otherwise noted on page 280
Interior design: Ralph Fowler
Editors: Shelly Antol, Andrea Vinley Jewell, Jim Ruark

Printed in the United States of America

14 15 16 17 18 19 /DCI/ 17 16 15 14 13 12 11 10 9 8 7 6 5 4 3 2 1

Medical Disclaimer

The Daniel Plan offers health, fitness, and nutritional information
and is for educational purposes only. This book is intended to
supplement, not replace, the professional medical advice, diag-
nosis, or treatment of health conditions from a trained health
professional. Please consult your physician or other healthcare
professional before beginning or changing any health or fitness
program to make sure that it is appropriate for your needs —
especially if you are pregnant or have a family history of any
medical concerns, illnesses, or risks.

    If you have any concerns or questions about your health,
you should always consult with a physician or other healthcare
professional. Stop exercising immediately if you experience faint-
ness, dizziness, pain, or shortness of breath at any time. Please
do not disregard, avoid, or delay obtaining medical or health-
related advice from your healthcare professional because of
something you may have read in this guide.

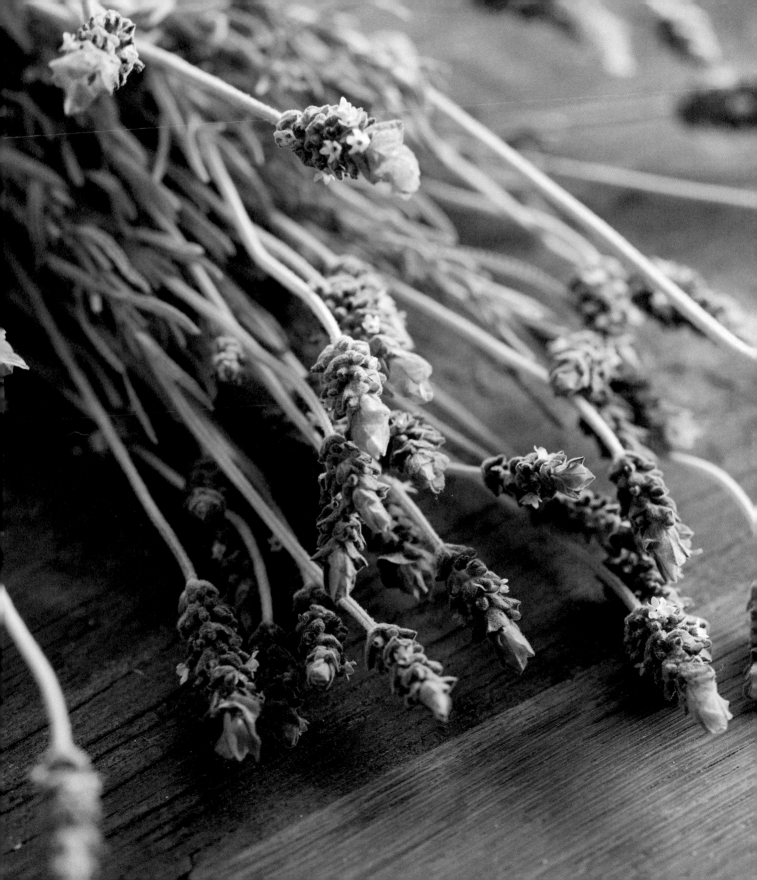

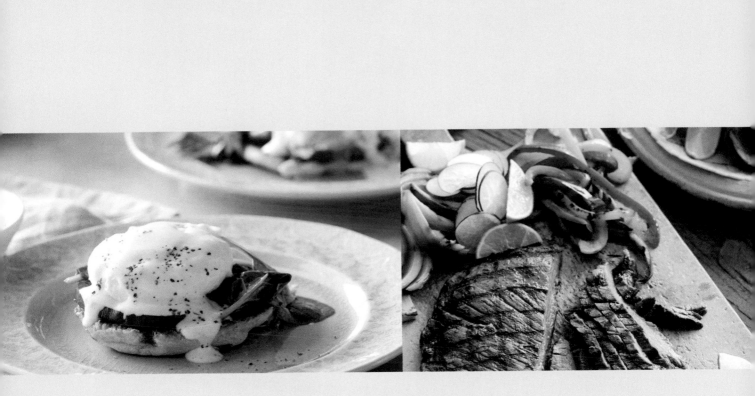

Contents

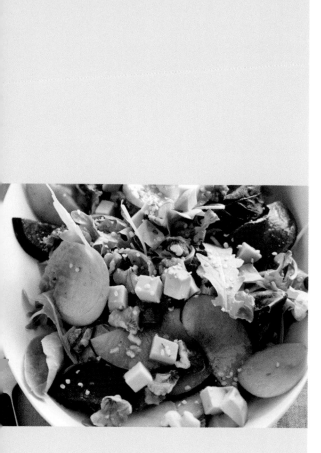

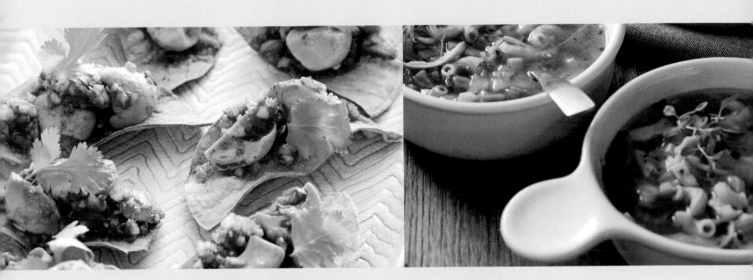

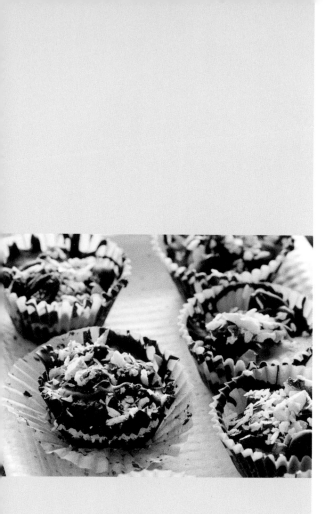

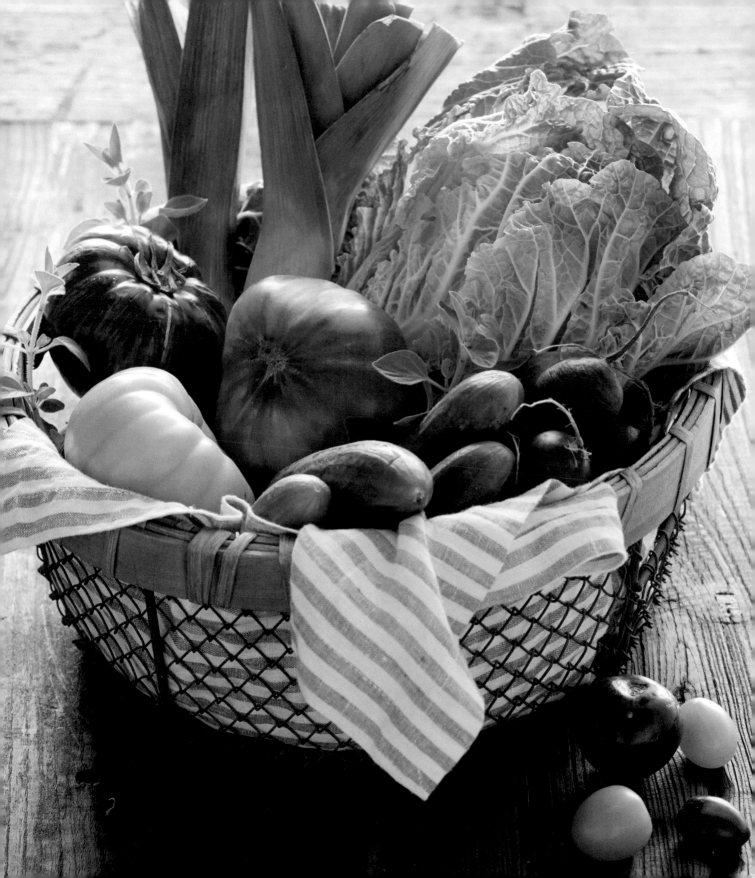

The Daniel Plan Approach to Healthy Eating for Life

*T*he Daniel Plan Cookbook is based on the Essentials written about in *The Daniel Plan: 40 Days to a Healthier Life*. The foundational principle for Daniel Plan eating is one of abundance, not deprivation. This is not a diet; it's a plan that you adopt for the rest of your life. It's a new way to live.

When you focus on eating The Daniel Plan way, health, healing, weight loss, balance, and increased energy are the natural result.

Food truly is medicine, and learning to cook is invaluable for your health. Food becomes a powerful healing force when you cook and eat whole, unprocessed, fresh foods made by God. So let's dive into Daniel Plan cooking.

American Classics, Made Healthy

For this cookbook we have created more than a hundred delicious, healthy recipes, transforming some of our favorite dishes. They are full of flavor, yet packed with benefits for your body. These wonderful foods taste good and promote a long and healthy life. We have also included tips for a Daniel Plan pantry and kitchen, plus tips on how to shop, plan menus, save time, prepare ahead, and snack smartly.

Maybe this is your first brave foray into the world of cooking. Maybe you are a seasoned home chef. Wherever your cooking skills fall on this spectrum, we have created delicious, easy recipes to make mealtime enjoyable for everyone.

We began by thinking about you and what most people like to eat. We then created versions that fit with The Daniel Plan. Included are American classics such as burgers, tacos and meatloaf, soups, salads, and stews. We created great recipes for chicken, beef, and fish as well as meatless dishes. Of course, you will find lots of vegetables, side dishes, and fabulous sauces. We have got you covered from breakfast and appetizers to snacks and dessert.

Read more about The Daniel Plan at *danielplan.com.*

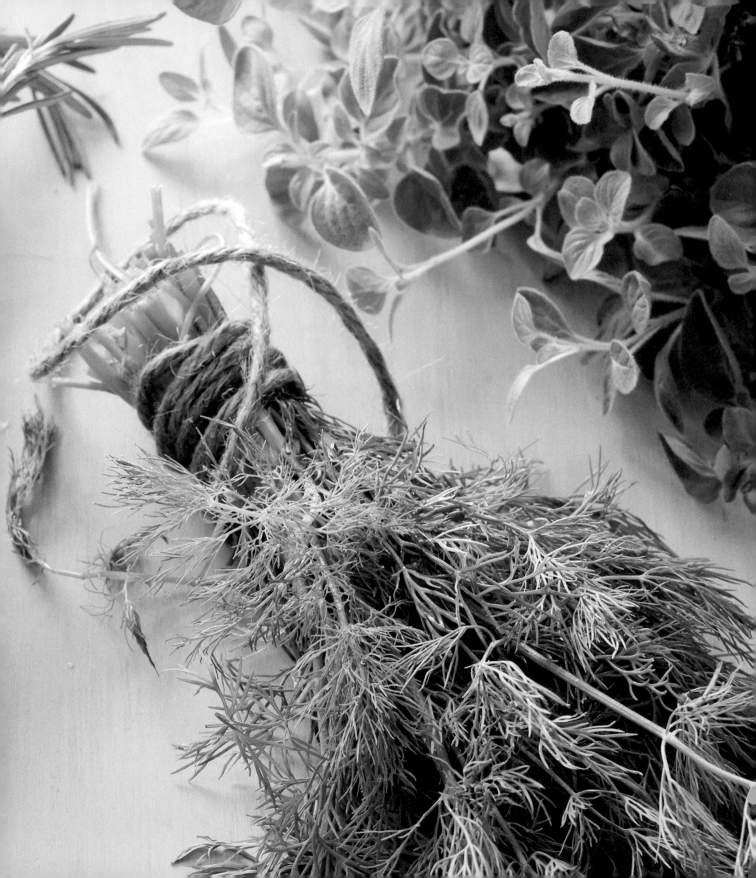

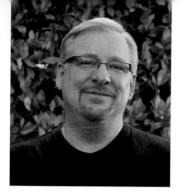

A Note from Pastor Rick Warren

On a typical summer morning when I was growing up, I would find my mom in the kitchen preparing all sorts of fruits and vegetables that we had picked from our garden. We lived on five acres, and my dad was an organic farmer before organic farming became an "in-thing."

As a sixth grader, I remember reading his monthly *Organic Gardening* magazine.

My mom always cooked with fresh ingredients straight from the garden. She would can, pickle, and freeze foods such as corn and strawberries and give away the rest.

As a result, one of my favorite things to do now is gather my kids and grandkids to cook and grill fresh food from our garden. Last year, even as a busy pastor, I grew fifty-eight varieties of vegetables and ten varieties of fruit trees. There is nothing better than homemade salsa and grilled veggies that were just picked

Over the years, gardening not only has provided our family with fresh, nutritious food, but has also cultivated my appreciation for what God provides. God's intention from the beginning (see Genesis 1:29) was to provide us with real, whole food—the

kind of food that allows us to stay healthy and live fully. God loves variety, and I see that in the abundant harvest of seasonal fruits and vegetables we get to enjoy.

When Kay and I got married, we were a great match because, for one thing, I love to eat and she loves to cook. Kay is an incredible baker, and in this cookbook you will see some of our family favorites.

In this cookbook you will find a menu of American classics that don't compromise taste and that will help you live healthier and give you energy to fulfill your God-given purpose. Food is one of the great ways to create fellowship and build relationships. So gather your friends and family and enjoy each other around the table. Get back in your kitchen, and rediscover how easy it is to cook fresh, delicious whole foods. God bless you.

Kitchen Talk with Dr. Amen & Dr. Hyman

Pastor Warren recruited three nationally known doctors — Daniel Amen, M.D.; Mark Hyman, M.D.; and Mehmet Oz, M.D. — to coach him in getting healthy and help design The Daniel Plan. All three doctors graciously volunteered their expertise and time for free because they care about our health. Dr. Hyman and Dr. Amen have transformed thousands of lives with their medical insight. Their passion to help people get well started years ago and affected their own lives. Get to know a little bit about their journey toward health and the impact that eating and cooking well has had on both of them.

What was the turning point for you that changed how you eat?

Dr. Amen: When I read the study that showed that as your weight went up the size of your brain went down, it just horrified me. I knew my brain was one of my most precious resources.

For thirty years I had been trying to lose weight. So when I got really serious about changing my eating habits, the big surprise for me was that I wasn't hungry. I took out the high-glycemic foods and got my vitamin D level normal. (It was 17 when I started, while normal is between 30 and 100). Plus, I realized that you actually have to eat to lose weight, but eating well got my appetite under control.

Dr. Hyman: I visited my sister at her college when I was fifteen years old, and she introduced me to the "veggie" room in her cafeteria. That's when I learned about crunchy organic peanut butter — rich, deep, and flavorful — slathered onto dense multi-grain homemade bread. The vegetarian food was so good, so delicious, that I became a vegetarian for eight years.

Then, in college I lived in a community house with eight people. Each of us cooked for everyone else one night a week. Making fresh, delicious, and inexpensive meals

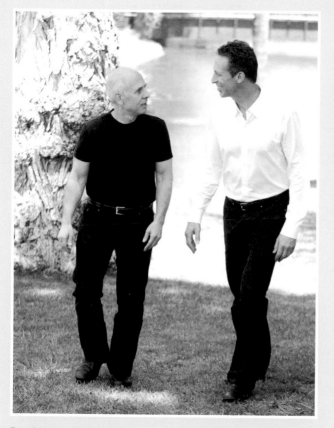

Dr. Amen and Dr. Hyman visit one of Saddleback Church's campuses.

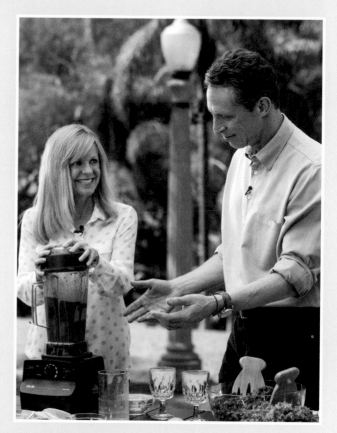

Dr. Hyman demonstrates one of his favorite smoothies for Daniel Plan Director Dee Eastman.

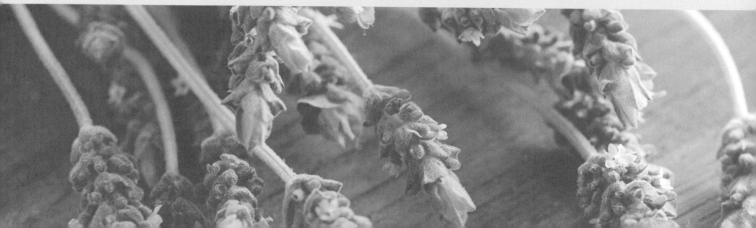

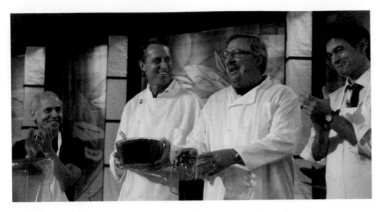

Dr. Amen, Dr. Hyman, Pastor Warren, and Dr. Oz
at the first Daniel Plan rally

from scratch (we had little money) for a bunch of hungry college students, and sharing the joy and pleasure of real food made with love was the beginning of a lifelong passion.

How have your eating choices changed your life?

Dr. Amen: In every way. If I am more conscious about my eating, I am also more conscious about my overall health and brain. If I am conscious about my eating, I am also more conscious about how I feed my loved ones. If I am conscious about my eating, I am now more conscious about the health of our planet and how agriculture affects many aspects of life.

Dr. Hyman: I love food. I eat almost anything, as long as it is made by God, not man. Food is the fabric that ties everything together for me — my health, my work, my family, my friends, and the health of our environment, even our global, social, and economic prosperity. Food is the medicine I use to treat my patients. It is more powerful than anything else I have at my disposal as a doctor to prevent, treat, and even reverse disease. Think about that the next time you take a bite of something.

How long did it take for your food tastes to change?

Dr. Amen: Literally less than two weeks. It was more my mind that had to change. When I realized that I was loving to eat right, what was good for me tasted a whole lot better.

Dr. Hyman: It took one week for me. Once you unhook from processed food, sugar, flour, and industrial packaged foods, your taste buds change, your brain chemistry gets reset, and you quickly stop craving the junk and start craving vegetables — really!

Dr. Amen: You should see us [Dr. Hyman, Dr. Oz, and me] when we are together: we're like squirrels. We take healthy food with us wherever we go; we stash it in our desks, our pockets, and our briefcases. That's how vigilant we are about healthy eating.

What are some foods that you used to love that you can't imagine eating today?

Dr. Amen: Brownies, Snickers, Rocky Road ice cream, pancakes, muffins …

simple carbohydrates that boost the risk of diabetes and Alzheimer's disease. For me, I have to be really careful, because I can easily get triggered to dive back into those foods. So I am irritatingly vigilant for the health of my brain and my body. My treat is 65 percent dark chocolate that has DHA [an omega–3 fatty acid] in it. Eating well means there is no suffering required.

Dr. Hyman: When I was a kid, I loved Twinkies, Hostess Cup Cakes, Lik-m-aid, Smarties, and Peanut M&Ms. I used to pour powdered colored flavored sugar into my mouth. Now my body rejects those things. I walk by the candy aisle, and no matter how hungry I am, it just doesn't register as food. In fact, when I eat food-like substances, my body now knows immediately. I get sores in my mouth, my tongue feels weird, and I get a strange cloudy feeling in my head. So I can't imagine eating junk or candy; I love the naturally sweet things — fruit, maple syrup, honey.

For someone just starting, what important first steps would you suggest?

Dr. Amen: Prayer, education, motivation, support, and brain envy. It all comes down to our minds and what we believe about ourselves. If you start today, think about what your life will be like in thirty or sixty or ninety days. Then think about what your life will be like ninety days from now if you don't change your health. If you are like most people who start The Daniel Plan, you will feel better, your clothes will be loose, and you will have to go shopping.

Dr. Hyman: I agree. The first step in changing how you eat is to connect to why you want to change. Once you realize you want to change, I recommend a very short detox. It can be a powerful way to realize just how bad the food you were eating truly makes you feel, and how quickly and easily you can feel better. It is also important to design your life for success. Clean up your pantry. Put real food in your kitchen. Stock emergency food packs so you always have something to eat that will nourish you.

When you cook, what are the go-to ingredients that you have to have on hand?

Dr. Amen: Tana—my wife! When I met her, she didn't know how to cook. I didn't even want her to cook! She would make a mess in the kitchen. But as she became more familiar with my work, and because she had cancer that came back three times, she began to take health seriously. So she figured out how to become masterful at taking healthy foods and making them taste great.

Besides Tana, in our kitchen we always have lean protein powder, frozen berries, spinach, and sugar-free dark chocolate.

Dr. Hyman: I stock my kitchen so that even if I don't have time to shop or plan, I always have something to eat or can make a simple meal in less than thirty minutes. I was recently gone for three weeks, but when I got home, I was able to cook a delicious meal from scratch from the foods I had on hand. Buying a few fresh vegetables on my way home from work once or twice a week allows me to make a simple meal anytime.

Do you have any tips for getting kids involved with cooking?

Dr. Amen: Cook with them. Give them skills, and let them have success with healthy food.

Dr. Hyman: Make it fun. Put on fun music in the kitchen. Dance and sing in the kitchen so they have good memories of being there. When my children were little, we made cooking a family adventure. Children naturally love to help, to play with food and learn. So bake with them. Teach them to chop vegetables. Make a pie. Teach them how to grill ribs or make shish kebabs.

Dr. Amen: Tana and I cook with my grandkids. One of my grandchildren came to live with us for six months. We would cook with her, and she learned how to cook healthy food. My daughter, who is ten, spends a lot of time in the kitchen with her mom. She is so proud of herself because she can make a totally healthy pumpkin spice cake. One of my grandkids helps herself to the shelf in our pantry that has all kinds of ingredients for smoothies and shakes — she makes her own. If we make them teachers, then they teach their friends and families.

Dr. Hyman: Why not grow a small garden and allow them to plant, weed, water, and harvest their food so they have a real connection to where food comes from? Take kids shopping. Teach them to choose real food, such as how to know if a vegetable is fresh or a fruit is ripe, or how to shop from a recipe. Make it a family event.

Tell us one of your favorite meals and who you shared it with?

Dr. Amen: Tana and I were traveling together in Texas and went out for dinner. We ate Cioppiono, grass-fed New York steak, sautéed spinach, and asparagus. It was amazing! I looked at her and said, "This is not really suffering." Eating well is about believing that you are worth it and that you are more valuable than your cravings.

Dr. Hyman: Every summer I go to Cape Cod for vacation with my family and friends. We have a tradition of a seafood feast with lobster, steamed local clams, fresh summer corn on the cob, a big salad of summer tomatoes, arugula, and avocados. We make a mess and laugh and tell stories on the deck outside.

How do you plan out your meals for the week? Any tips?

Dr. Amen: I say, "Fail to plan, then plan to fail." We get together at the beginning of the week and decide what we will eat for dinners. Breakfast is usually a protein shake, and lunch can be sushi or a chicken salad or stir-fry minus the rice.

Dr. Hyman: I make it simple. I have one or two breakfasts, one or two lunches, and three to four dinners that I can whip up quickly. I save the more elaborate recipes and meals for special occasions or weekends when I have more time. For breakfast I stick with my whole foods protein shake (page 76) or a couple of eggs, poached or lightly fried in olive oil, and an avocado. For lunch I have salad with avocado, toasted nuts, cherry tomatoes, arugula, and a can of wild salmon on top. For dinner: grilled chicken or fish, or sautéed tofu, stir-fried broccoli, asparagus or broccoli rabe or broccolini in olive oil with a little mirin (Japanese rice wine), salt, and pepper. I make some black rice for the week and store it in the fridge, then just reheat it in a pan.

What is the one health tip you tell people that has profoundly changed your life?

Dr. Amen: I always ask myself, *Then what?* If I eat this, then what? How will I feel in thirty–sixty minutes? How will I look next week or next month?

Dr. Hyman: Have protein for breakfast. Every day. No exceptions. Protein is a powerful way to start the day and is a key to weight loss and health.

How do you create healthy mealtime celebrations for birthday, holidays, and family gatherings?

Dr. Amen: Often people celebrate with food that makes us sick. They soothe others with food or drink that is bad for us. So in my house, we create brain-healthy treats instead: fruit plates, nuts, fresh no-sugar-added sorbets (fruit has enough sugar), and frozen bananas.

Dr. Hyman: The happiest times for me are inviting friends and family over and cooking a fabulous (but often simple) meal for us all to share and enjoy together. We go to the garden together and pick our dinner. Or they help cut veggies or just hang out in the kitchen with good music playing in the background. Building family traditions around food is a wonderful way to create happy memories and build lifelong connections with family and friends.

The Daniel Plan Detox

Pick up a copy of *The Daniel Plan: 40 Days to a Healthier Life* for more information on the detox meal plan to reset your body and your tastes.

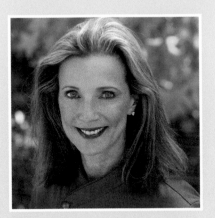

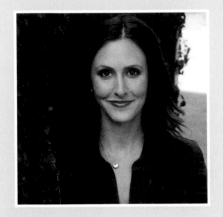

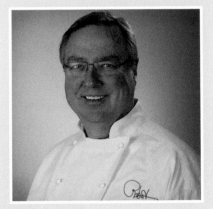

Sally Cameron

Jenny Ross

Robert Sturm

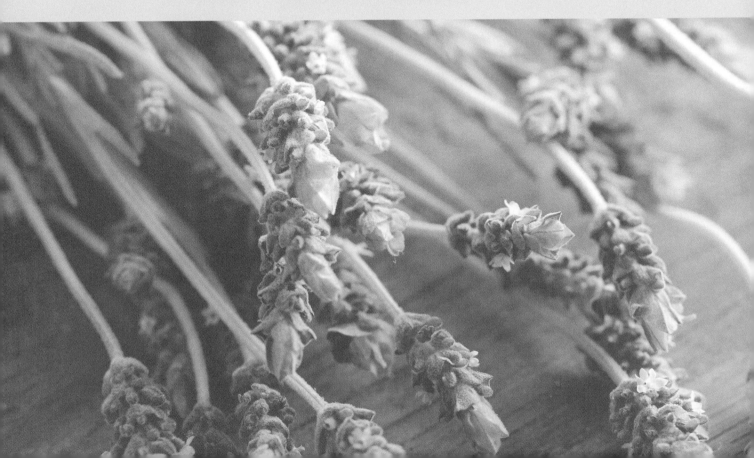

The Daniel Plan
Signature Chefs

The Daniel Plan Signature Chefs developed, created, cooked, tested, and did it all over again and again to create delicious, nutritious recipes made from real whole foods and ingredients.

Sally Cameron is a professional chef, certified health coach, speaker, and author. Sally's passion is to inspire people to create great-tasting meals at home using healthy ingredients and easy techniques. Sally is the publisher of the popular food blog A Food Centric Life. Sally works with clients, including professional athletes and public figures, to help them achieve their individual health goals through optimum food choices and culinary and nutritional coaching. She holds a culinary degree from The Art Institute and health coaching certification from The Institute for Integrative Nutrition.

Jenny Ross is an internationally recognized chef, author, and educator, and the force behind Jenny Ross Living Foods, including the raw food restaurants 118 Degrees, the popular Raw Basics detox meal programs, and nationwide grocery product

line 118 Degrees. She has been an early pioneer of the raw movement, coaching clients about the healing power of living foods, while motivating them to adopt a more vibrant, healthy lifestyle. Find more about raw food in *Healing with Raw Foods, Raw Basics, Simply Dehydrated* or *The Art of Raw Living Food* cookbooks. She has a degree in holistic nutrition and certificates as a health and life coach.

Robert Sturm is one of California's premier chefs and food designers. He has been in the food service industry for more than thirty years, working as an independent consultant to leading restaurant chains around the country. He has been featured in many publications, appears on television and radio, and has been a featured chef at the United Nations, the White House, and the Kremlin.

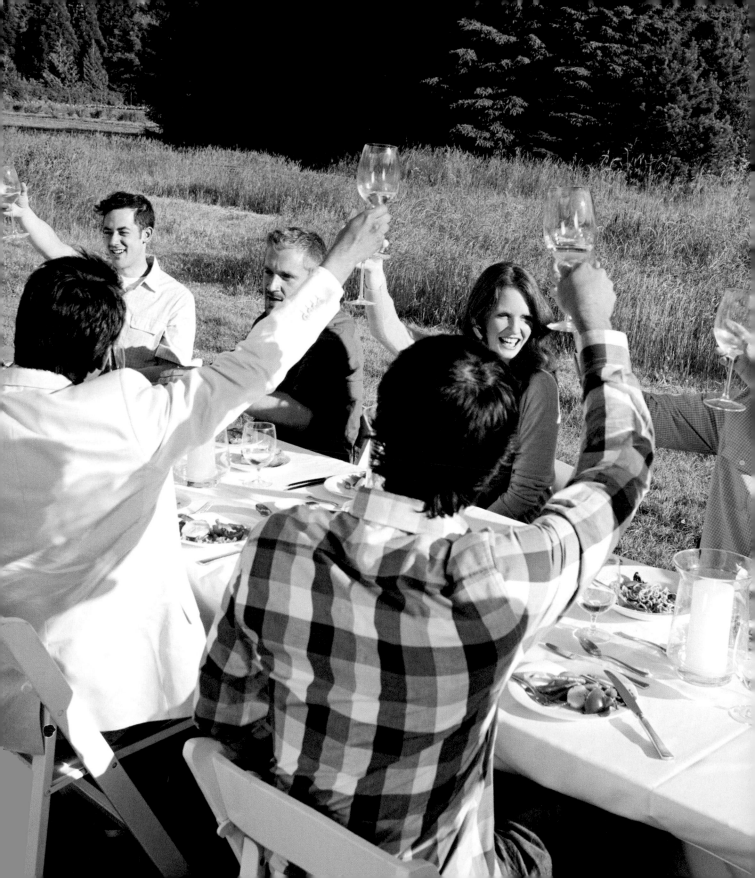

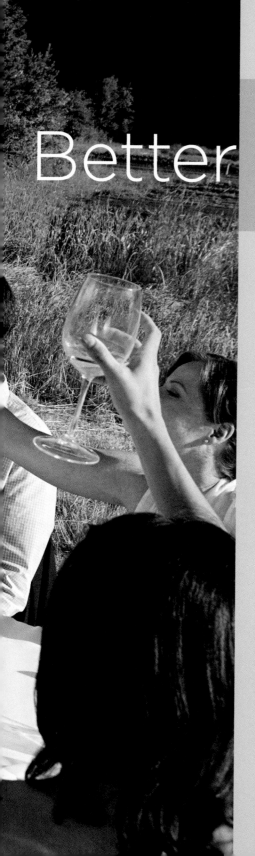

Better Together

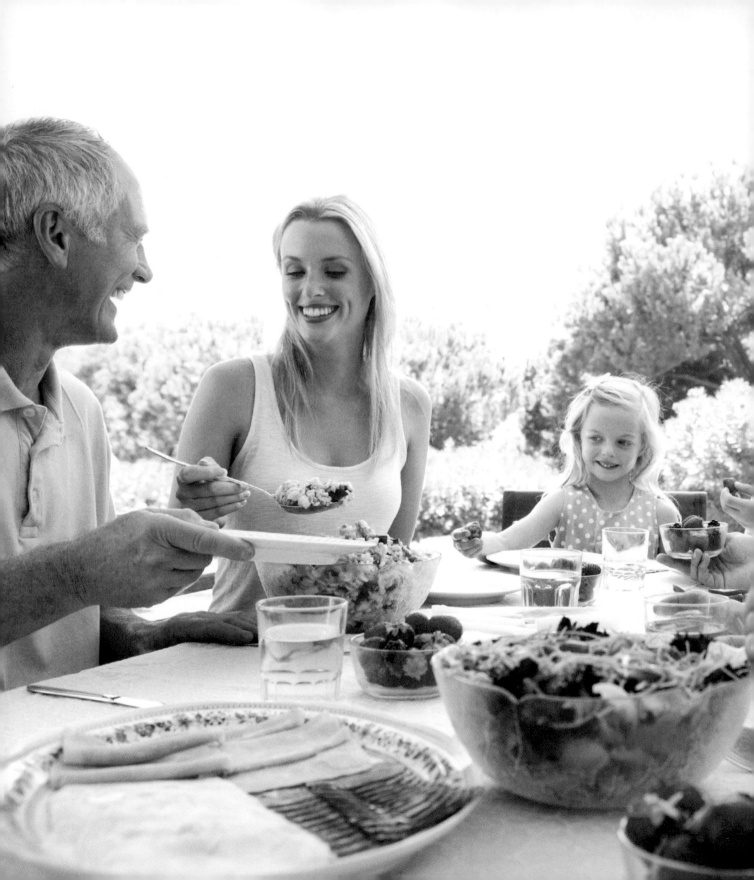

Gather Around
The Daniel Plan Table

If we told you that you could be two to three times more successful on The Daniel Plan, would you want to know how? We would! The "secret sauce"— as we like to call it—is friends. It's that simple.

We are better together, and The Daniel Plan is proof that our friends help transform our lives—even when it comes to our physical health. A community that offers support and inspiration keeps you moving forward toward a healthier life.

One of the oldest pastimes is gathering for meals at a communal table. Humans have been hunting, gathering, and eating together for centuries. Families eat together. Kings and queens feast. Warring tribes agree to treaties over meals. We celebrate and find comfort around food. Around the dining table and kitchen, we can cheer our successes, commiserate about our challenges, and encourage one another. What a perfect place to also focus on our health!

The more people you can share The Daniel Plan with, the more you will find success with and enjoyment of your food choices. So while this cookbook is all about giving you the tools to cook healthy real food, we invite you to do it with others. Make dinner together, share recipes, plan potlucks, and explore new foods with your friends and family.

In the simple process of meeting together over food, your ideas of "social eating" will begin to shift toward healthier choices. One group of friends who were discovering The Daniel Plan together started including and focusing on healthy foods at each get-together. After several weeks on The Daniel Plan, more than 80 percent of the group had marked improvements in their health. Two individuals got off blood pressure medications, one member met her weight goal, and another member reported an increased level of energy and vitality after eliminating coffee from his diet.

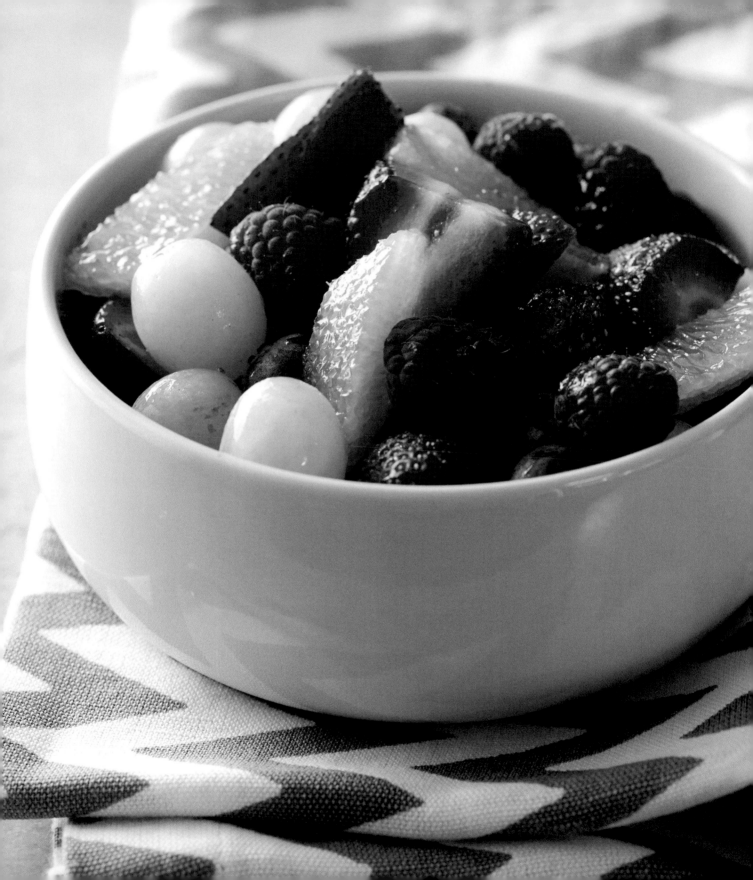

These friends supported each other between meetings by calling one another throughout the week, sharing success stories, asking for help, and encouraging one another after natural slip-ups or unhealthy choices. Their tastes changed, and they started craving foods that are good for them. To infuse fun learning into their journey, they even invited a local health foods chef to demo a few Daniel Plan recipes for their whole group. Together they discovered new food items and learned cooking tips.

The secret sauce of community can come from your own family, coworkers, neighbors, or small groups. You may be inspired or called to lead your own group of Daniel Plan participants. Leading others into The Daniel Plan lifestyle can be as simple as sharing the fun and fulfilling recipes from this cookbook at the next neighborhood block party and being open about your own health journey. If you love cooking already, you could be a health champion and show others the ropes in the kitchen.

Some basic things you might try with friends or family: Share a healthy meal each week, each of you bringing a dish that you enjoy; visit local health workshops; or attend culinary classes geared toward wellness. Potlucks, parties, and make-your-own dinners get everyone involved in the kitchen, while also promoting health and the joy of shared meals.

Ultimately, the secret sauce is the one ingredient we want you to use over and over. The power of two or more can remind you of how far you have come on The Daniel Plan and provide tangible inspiration as you continue on your journey.

Share a Meal

For more great ideas on how to set the "community table" on The Daniel Plan, check out Mealtime Celebrations on pages 250 – 263.

Turn Ordinary Moments into Special Moments

Sitting down to eat a meal together around the table is a great time to learn how everyone is doing. Whether you are enjoying a meal with friends on the weekend or sitting down to a family supper during the week, mealtimes help people stay connected. With demanding schedules and a multitude of activities, it's easy to see why plans to eat together can often get derailed. But shared meals are a practice you will want to preserve. Consider a meal a date with your loved ones, a reservation that reveals how much you care.

Take time at the table for everyone to share about what's happening at school or work and talk about upcoming events. It's a chance to listen and an opportunity to be heard. One approach that gets things started is called "highs and lows." Each person talks about a high point and a low point of the day or week. Letting each person open up in this way often leads to deeper conversations. Then go around the table and affirm each other. You will be surprised how much you learn during just one meal!

Once a week or month, set the table for a party to celebrate milestones and special

Family, Food, and Kids

The latest research shows that kids, especially teenagers, are less likely to get lured into trouble and experiment with drugs if they eat regularly with their family. The family bonding and support also fosters their academic life. Kids who go to school hungry don't learn as well. A hearty breakfast is a must for everyone.

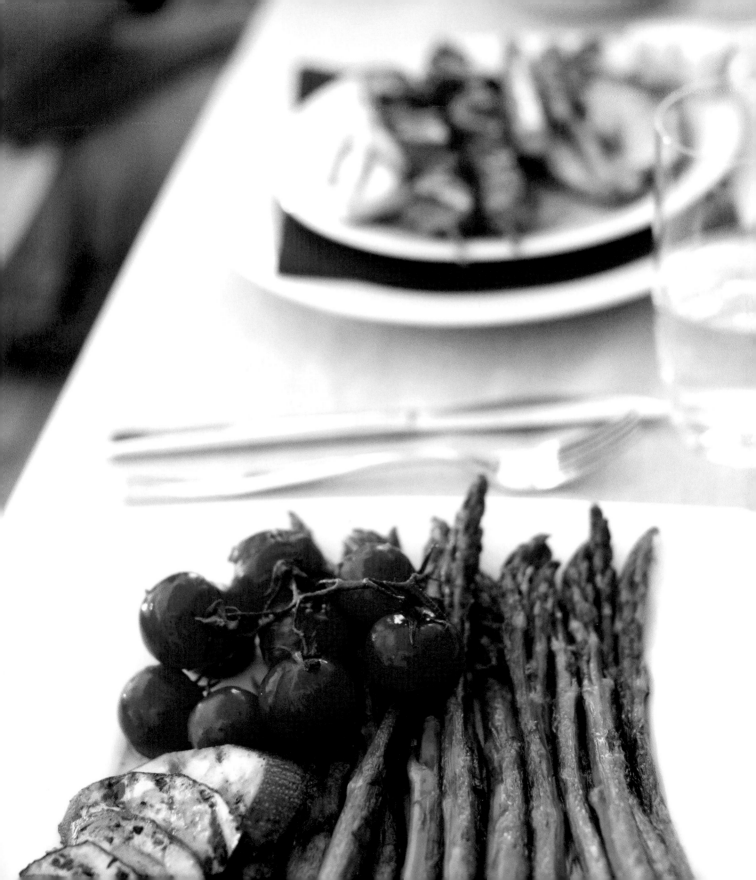

achievements. Designate a special plate or table decorations for the occasion. When you stop to think about it, there is always something to celebrate besides the big events of a birthday, graduation, or anniversary. Recognize an accomplishment at work or school, a deadline that was met, a new skill learned, an answered prayer, or a new friend made. Celebrating together is a joy generator. With a life full of commitments and obligations, isn't it nice to welcome a little bliss whenever we can?

Take the leap. Set a schedule and send out the invitation. You will wonder why you didn't do it sooner. It's just a healthy way to nurture the ones you love. At some point, take it a step further and invite others to join your family, perhaps a friend who lives alone, a neighbor who has recently divorced, or anyone who could use some loving care. Hospitality offers comfort and acceptance to whoever accepts the invitation. Open your door and your heart to share your meals and moments around the table. You will likely be inspired to make it an ongoing tradition.

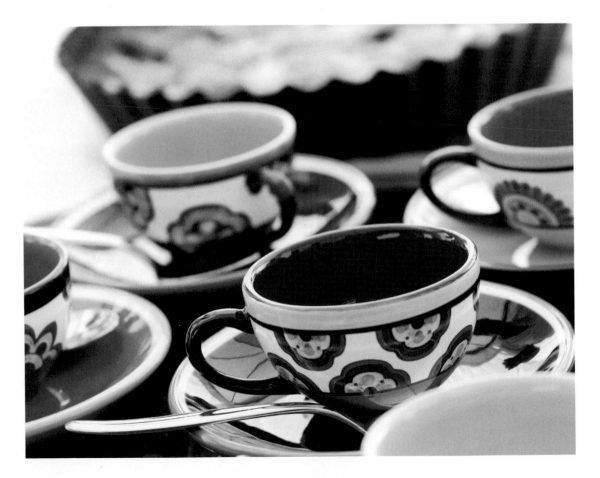

The Family Kitchen

Naturally, you may be wondering exactly how you will engage your children, older family members, and maybe even your spouse in The Daniel Plan menu. Anyone who has children knows that change in the dinner time routine can be a source of conflict and stress. Just dining in can be a new concept for your family, especially if you have a busy schedule. To avoid this, we recommend planning ahead.

The most important thing you can share as you begin to discover real, whole foods together is the reason behind the change. Families who are united for better health can create a foundation for a well-balanced life. Take the time to talk about why health is important. Encourage everyone to take The Daniel Plan as a family exploration adventure. It's okay that not everyone will like every option; don't let it be a downer or source of tension. Instead, make it fun by encouraging everyone to be adventurous and try everything at least once. You might consider posting a food ranking chart in your kitchen or dining room and ask everyone to offer two to three words to describe the flavor and texture of foods — even if those descriptions are the reason they don't like something.

Kids of all ages can become Daniel Plan chefs. When family members encourage them, many children are excited about the prospect of creating something in the kitchen. Kids in particular display a proud sense of ownership for meals they create, so engage them in food preparations as often as possible — and be patient with them.

Starting on page 15 we talk about some easy ways to plan ahead and organize your kitchen with the basic ingredients for making quick and easy Daniel Plan meals throughout the week. Kids and teens can help by labeling containers, washing vegetables, and having shopping duties. With your strong readers, consider putting them on a "search and destroy" mission in the pantry to help you clean it out. Love

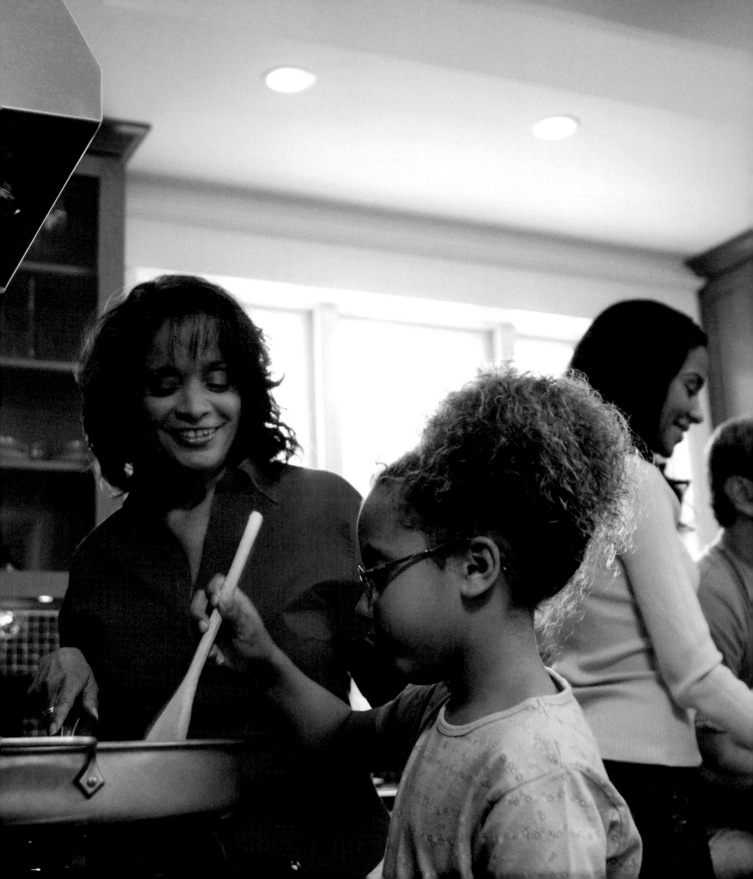

of good food begins with picking out the ingredients, so involve your children in all steps of the process for best results and a long-lasting relationship with healthy food.

We also have a few tricks for helping family members get some important Daniel Plan basics into their diet. For greens, we recommend smoothies such as the Green Smoothie on page 79. It looks green, but does not taste "green." For fruits and vegetables, we recommend plating them in interesting ways. We eat with our eyes first, so the more interesting the food looks, the more likely we are to be willing to try it. Here are a few ideas:

- The Zucchini Pasta on page 113 can be served piled high using a compression mold to stack the pasta and create a tower. Your little ones might have even more fun by adding castle windows and doors, using baby tomatoes.

- Instead of tossing or layering salads, arrange items to create shapes and characters (e.g., tomato for a head, lettuce for a body, carrots for arms and legs). There are reasons why fun pasta and cereal shapes sell! Put those kid-friendly tactics to work in your kitchen.

- Occasionally set up interactive family meals, such as creating a salad, taco, or sandwich bar where family members can add their favorite toppings to healthy basics.

As you explore your Daniel Plan preferences with your family, you may experience certain meal-planning challenges when accommodating a variety of food restrictions in your family. View this as an opportunity for the whole family to try new versions of certain dishes. For example, if one family member is lactose intolerant, have the entire family show their support by choosing a dairy-free meal each week. As you model healthy habits and supportive choices at the dinner table, your children will begin to see the table as a safe and fun place for health and family time.

A little creativity can go a long way toward inspiring health for the whole family. For more ideas on creative family expressions of The Daniel Plan, check out our Facebook page with ongoing posts on creative Daniel Plan feasts for the whole family.

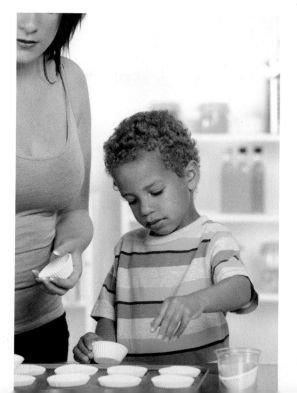

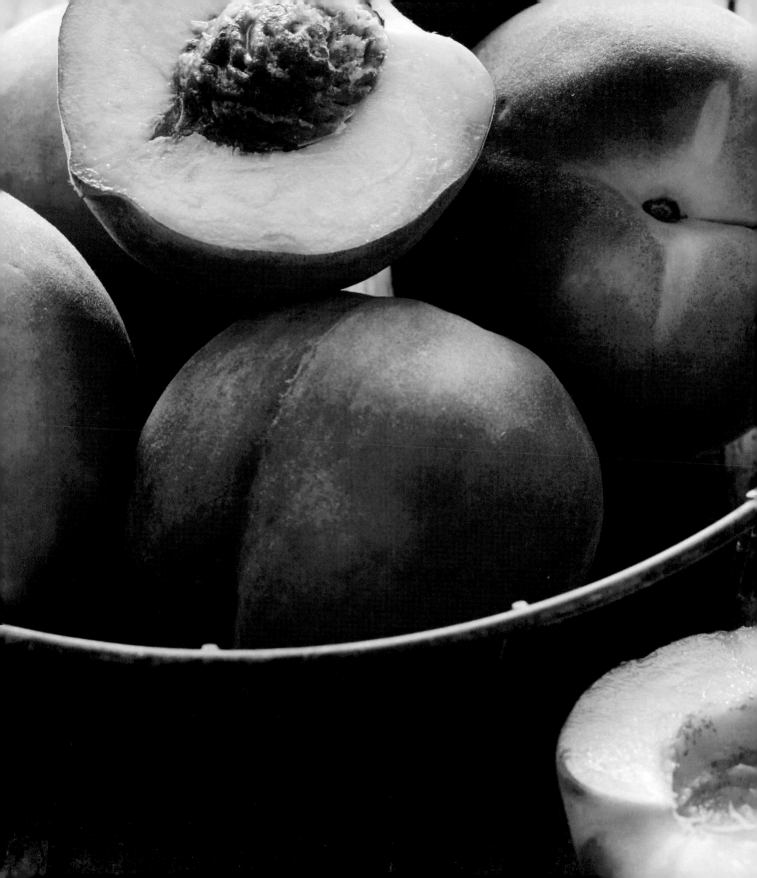

Getting Started

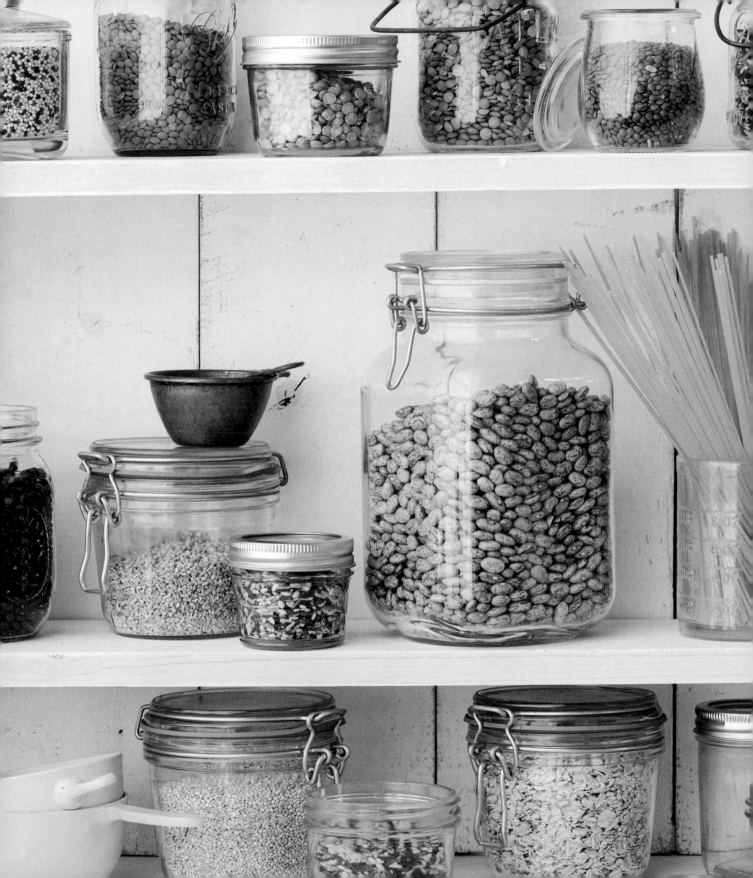

Creating a
Daniel Plan Pantry

Out with the old and in with the new! The first step in creating a Daniel Plan pantry is to clean out the stuff that is not serving you well. This means reading labels, checking expiration dates, tossing or donating the bad stuff, then refilling with healthful new items.

While we want you to focus on the abundance of delicious whole foods, we also want you to know what harmful foods to remove from your pantry and shopping lists for good. Simply getting rid of these foods from your eating life will make a tremendous difference in your health and eating habits.

Do this with your dry pantry, where you store canned goods, whole grains, and nonperishables. While you are at it, go through your refrigerator and freezer, too, and toss things that have harmful ingredients.

Having good foods in your pantry will support healthy eating and save you time. With a well-stocked pantry, you will never be at a loss for something healthy to eat.

Choose a weekend to clean out the pantry, and make it a group project. Or choose a friend, and help each other do a pantry clean-out. Have a pantry clean-out party!

You might even treat yourself to a few new storage containers for bulk items you will be adding, such as brown and black rice, quinoa, and dried beans. Keep a pen and masking tape handy to label containers, or use a label-making tool. Be sure storage containers are clear so that you can see inside and make sure lids fit tight.

A few pantry clean-out tips:

- Read labels and check for unhealthy ingredients.

- Say good-bye to the "white menaces," as well as the things hiding in your pantry that are made with them.

- Banish processed foods such as sugary breakfast cereals, unhealthy cookies and crackers, fried chips, and junk food.

- Exile high-sugar or high-sodium condiments. (Read that ketchup bottle — you might be surprised.) Shop for healthier versions, comparing labels for ingredients.

- Evict unhealthy oils, such as standard mass-market "vegetable" oil. We will tell you what the good stuff is as you read further (page 47).

- Aim for labels with five ingredients or less or at least ingredients that you recognize as real food. If you don't understand what something is and your grandmother would not know what it is, it's probably not what you want in your pantry.

- As for those jars of dried herbs that look as if they have been around since the Stone Age — toss them. Do the same for old spices. When you open new containers, be sure to date them. More tips on herbs and spices are to come (page 43).

Easy Replacements and Alternatives

Reading through this list may feel overwhelming at first, but the good news is that for every harmful food or ingredient, there is a healthy, tasty alternative. We want you to pack your kitchen and pantry with so many good foods that will keep you satisfied that they crowd out the bad ones. Soon you will be an expert at choosing healthy alternatives to harmful foods and ingredients. And as your health and well-being improve, you will enjoy making better choices for the benefits they bring.

Foods and Ingredients to Avoid

White flour	White sugar	White rice
High fructose corn syrup (HFCS)	Trans fats, hydrogenated and partially hydrogenated fats	Monosodium glutamate (MSG)
Regular and diet sodas	Sports drinks and other sweetened beverages	Juice
Soy protein isolate	Sodium and calcium caseinate	Phosphoric acid
Artificial sweeteners (except stevia)	Artificial flavors	Artificial colors and dyes
Sulfites	Nitrites and nitrates	Carrageenan

Replace This	With This
Mass market vegetable oil	Unrefined, cold-pressed, and expeller-pressed oils such as extra-virgin olive oil, grape seed oil, coconut oil, avocado oil, and sesame oil
Shortening	Coconut butter or oil
White flour	Whole grain wheat flour, organic sprouted flour, almond flour, gluten-free flour, or organic cornmeal
Sugary cereals	Old-fashioned oats, steel-cut oats, buckwheat, or kasha
Milk or cream (for lactose intolerant)	Coconut or almond milk
Crackers	Whole grain or brown rice crackers
Fried potato or corn chips	Baked corn, baked vegetable, or brown rice chips
Cream-based soups	Creamy bean-based soups, vegetable puree soups, and soups made with alternative healthy milks
White pasta	Whole grain, brown rice, buckwheat, shirataki, or quinoa pasta
White Rice	Brown or black rice, quinoa, barley
Table salt	Kosher or sea salt
White sugar	Raw honey, pure maple syrup, whole stevia extract*
Sugary snacks	Nuts, nut butters, dark chocolate, plain Greek yogurt with berries or a little honey
Gummy candies	Dried fruits (e.g., figs, dates)
Condiments and sauces with MSG or HFCS	Spices, vinegars, herbs, and naturally produced products with no added sugar
Chip dips	Guacamole, hummus, tzatziki, salsa
Fruit juice	Herbal teas, water with citrus wedges

*For baking, sugar alternatives do not react the same, so an equal swap may not work; the desserts section of this cookbook will provide you with some excellent recipes that use sugar alternatives appropriately.

Setting Up a Daniel Plan Kitchen

Essential Tools

Cooking can be as simple or as involved and creative as you want it to be. Cooking can mean learning quick, basic recipes to get healthy food on the table fast for busy nights. It can also be relaxing and fun, getting the whole family or friends involved for less-busy nights and weekends. It all comes down to finding methods to enjoy the wonderful taste of fresh, whole foods that nourish our bodies, minds, and spirits.

Having the right tools on hand will make it easier. We have created basic recommendations for what you will need to set up your Daniel Plan kitchen. Keep in mind the number of people you cook for. A family of two will have different needs than a family of six because of the quantity of food being prepared.

Where to Shop for Tools

You will find many places to shop for kitchen tools. Find a restaurant supply in your area. Many are open to the public. You can find good, professional quality tools at good prices. If you already like to cook, you will be the proverbial kid in the candy store at a restaurant supply shop.

Check stores such as Target, Wal-Mart, and Bed, Bath and Beyond. You will find almost anything you need at one of these shops. Of course, there are the big cooking stores such as Williams-Sonoma and Sur La Table, and the culinary world is available online, along with reviews you can read before making any purchase.

Cutlery (Knives)

Sharp knives actually make cooking easier and more efficient. While you may be tempted, do not buy a block full of knives at a big warehouse store. A few basic sizes will get you started.

Visit a store that carries knives, such as a cooking store or knife merchant. Hold various brands of knives in your hands. Get a feel for what is comfortable for you. Then get three knives: a 3-inch paring knife for small tasks, a 7-inch Santoku (a multi-purpose Japanese style knife) for general tasks, and an 8- to 9-inch chef's knife for larger tasks.

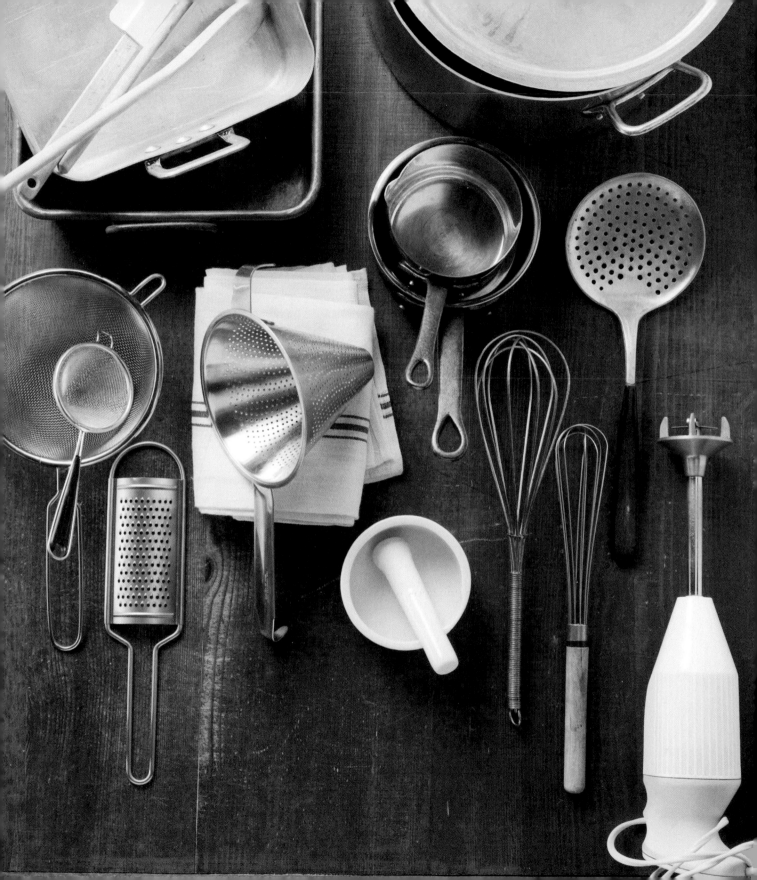

Good knives, when properly cared for, will last a lifetime. Store them in a wooden knife block or with plastic edge guards. After use, wash in dish soap and hot water, then dry with a kitchen towel. Never put knives in the dishwasher. It ruins the sharp edges. Several times a year, sharpen your knives with a sharpening steel or stone or at a knife shop.

Cutting Boards

Cutting boards come in a wide variety of materials, sizes, and price ranges. Be sure what you buy is food-safe. Nonporous, non-absorbent polypropylene cutting boards (which look like heavy thick plastic) and wooden cutting boards will not dull knives and are reversible. Polypropylene boards are generally dishwasher-safe. After repeated use, wooden cutting boards may get dry and should be oiled. Another option is a flexible, lightweight, nonporous cutting mat that bends so that you can pour ingredients into pan.

After use, rinse cutting boards and wash them with dish soap and hot water. Allow them to air dry or dry with a kitchen towel. For a lifetime of use, follow manufacturer's directions for care.

Cookware (Pots and Pans)

Available in many price ranges, quality pots and pans will help you to be more successful in cooking. Invest in heavy (versus lightweight) pots and pans, which distribute heat more evenly for better cooking and better results.

When buying pots and pans, what you purchase will depend on the task and how many people you generally cook for. All pans work on gas and electric stove tops. For induction cooktops, cookware will need to be magnetic or induction-approved.

Two-quart pots work for small jobs such as cooking rice and heating up smaller portions of things such as soup and sauces. The workhorses of your kitchen will be in the 4- to 5-quart range. If you cook for a larger family, you may need a pot or two in the 6- to 8-quart or larger range.

A 5½-quart enamel-coated cast iron Dutch Oven is a versatile pot and a nice size for soups, stews, and hearty sauces. This heavyweight cooks evenly at low temperatures on both the stove top and in the oven.

Larger pans with flat surfaces can be called sauté pans, fry pans, or skillets, depending on the manufacturer. Sides can

Chef's Trick

For keeping cutting boards from sliding on countertops: Place dampened paper towels or damp kitchen towels under the board for stability.

be flared or straight. Flared sides make for easier turning of food. Straight sides ease splattering and clean up. Good, useful sizes are 10- to 12-inch or 3- to 6-quart.

You will want a nonstick pan for cooking delicate things such as eggs or omelets, pancakes, and ingredients that tend to stick, such as burgers and seafood. Many of today's advanced non-stick surfaces can brown, sear, and withstand higher temperatures. When purchasing non-stick cookware, look for PFOA-free brands. They are safer for your family and the environment.

Small Electric Appliances

The two most important small appliances for a Daniel Plan kitchen are a blender and a food processor. Before you shop, read reviews online and check the details of what the models include. Don't bother with a mini food processor, as it is very limiting.

Other appliances: A handheld immersion blender is another handy tool for making sauces and for blending or pureeing right in a pan or pot. Some models come with whisk attachments. You might add a waffle iron or a Panini press, depending on what you love to cook and what your family loves to eat.

Small Tools

There are many small, inexpensive tools that will make prepping and cooking easier and faster. You probably own several of them already. For tools you do not own,

consider how often you might use them in your kitchen before buying them.

PFOA-free

- Wooden spoons and spatulas
- Flexible spatula (slotted metal) and turners
- Silicone, heat-proof spatulas and spoons
- Microplane or rasp zester and grater
- Garlic press
- Graduated measuring spoons
- Graduated dry measuring cups
- Liquid measuring cups
- Bamboo or metal skewers
- Mandoline or julienne slicing tool
- Handheld citrus press
- Vegetable peeler
- Digital thermometer (such as a Thermapen)
- Digital scale
- Tongs, metal and silicone-tipped
- Can opener
- Soft brush for scrubbing vegetables
- Colanders and strainers
- Mixing and prep bowls in graduated sizes
- Whisks, small and large
- Kitchen or poultry shears
- Rimmed baking sheets, quarter and half sizes

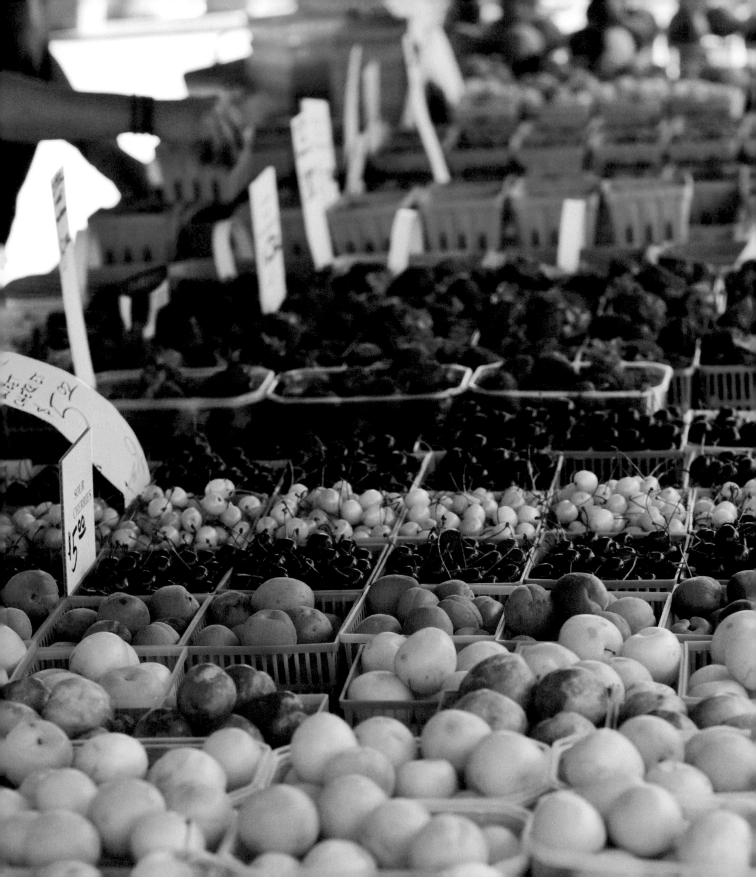

How to Shop Yourself Healthy

Where to Shop

If you think shopping is a chore, hopefully Daniel Plan shopping will change your mind! Whether you are at a farmers market; grocery, specialty, or health store; CSA (community-supported agriculture); food co-ops; or online, buying healthy ingredients that taste good can make you want to get into the kitchen and cook. And be sure to check out unique ethnic markets in your area for what they have to offer.

Buying fresh, locally grown, whole foods, fruits, vegetables, leafy greens, and sustainable meats and seafood is becoming easier for everyone across the country, thanks to the explosion of farmers markets and an increase of organic produce and healthy items available at mainstream grocers. Rest assured that your local grocery store will have most of what you need to start cooking and eating The Daniel Plan way. We will help you navigate the aisles and become a pro at shopping for your health.

Simple Shopping Tips

1. **Shop the perimeter.** The perimeter of the market is where the produce, eggs, meat, and seafood departments are located.

2. **Buy in bulk.** Many stores have a bulk area for non-perishable items such as rice and grains, dried beans, lentils and legumes, nuts, and seeds. Buying in bulk saves money.

3. **Brave the inside aisles.** Although there are many aisles you now can totally skip — which will save you time (and money!) — the inside aisles are where you will find packaged whole grains, canned beans, frozen berries and vegetables, healthy oils, vinegars, dried herbs and spices, packaged nuts, broths, and condiments.

4. **Keep it cool.** When you buy fresh seafood, ask for ice to keep it cold until you get home. Seafood is highly perishable. Use insulated shopping bags to help keep cold things cold. Have the store clerk pack all of your cold and frozen things together in one bag.

5. Stock up wisely. When nonperishable items such as grains, beans, boxed broth, and canned or jarred tomatoes are on sale, stock up and save money. Be smart about how much you can store and how much you will seriously use. This includes frozen items such as berries for smoothies and fresh, ground meat and poultry that will keep when wrapped well (or vacuum-sealed) in the freezer. Nuts, which can be expensive, store in the freezer for up to six months when wrapped well or vacuum-sealed.

If something looks like a great deal, it might be, but not always. Be sure to check expiration dates if an item is on sale—especially when buying oils, eggs, dairy, and other perishable items.

Chef's Trick

Cut the cooking instructions off the original packing for rice, legumes, and grains when you pour them into your storage containers. Then just set the instructions in the container for quick reference.

Learn to Read Labels

Learning to read labels or ingredients lists is an essential shopping skill (see examples on page 25). When you are buying fresh, whole foods such as fruits and vegetables, it is easy. You choose what is most fresh, smooth, ripe, crisp, and good.

But when you purchase pantry staples, such as canned beans, tomatoes, chicken or vegetable broth, and condiments, you must read labels to identify unhealthy ingredients.

Here is the skinny on ingredient labels:

- Ingredients are listed in descending order by proportion or quantity. So if the first item listed is beans, that is good. It means there are more beans than anything else in the can. If it is sugar, look for another option. Read the full ingredients list in any case, however, because culprits may be hiding lower in the list.

- Be wary of sodium levels, especially in broths and condiments. Compare labels and brands, and choose wisely.

- Aim for five ingredients or less. If ingredients sound as if they belong in a chemistry lab, pass.

- Do not believe health claims. They can be deceptive. If a label claims "trans fat free," it can still have trans fats. Companies are allowed to say a food is trans fat free if it has less than 0.5 grams in a serving. They get to round down and call it 0. Also, look for the terminology *partially hydrogenated*.

Granola Bar

INGREDIENTS: DRY ROASTED CASHEWS, DRY ROASTED ALMONDS, **BROWN RICE SYRUP,** SWEETENED CRANBERRIES (CRANBERRIES, **SUGAR,** SUNFLOWER OIL), **DRIED CANE SYRUP, DEXTROSE,** CRISP RICE (RICE FLOUR, **SUGAR,** SALT, MALT), PISTACHIOS, SWEETENED APRICOTS (APRICOTS, **SUGAR,** RICE FLOUR, CITRIC ACID), **HONEY, OAT SYRUP SOLIDS,** SEA SALT, ORANGE PEEL, SOY LECITHIN, ASCORBIC ACID (VITAMIN C) AND MIXED TOCOPHEROLS ADDED FOR FRESHNESS

- **Sugar** in many forms!

Salad Dressing

INGREDIENTS: TOMATO PUREE (WATER, TOMATO PASTE), **SUGAR,** WATER, VINEGAR, CORN SYRUP, CHOPPED PICKLES, **SOYBEAN OIL,** SALT, MODIFIED FOOD STARCH, CONTAINS LESS THAN 2% OF **XANTHAN GUM, ARTIFICIAL COLOR, PHOSPHORIC ACID, POLYSORBATE 60,** DRIED ONIONS, MUSTARD FLOUR, SPICE, GUAR GUM, **YELLOW 6, YELLOW 5, NATURAL FLAVOR,** OLEORESIN TURMERIC, POTASSIUM SORBATE AND CALCIUM DISODIUM EDTA (TO PROTECT FLAVOR)

- The second ingredient listed is **Sugar**, which means much of this product is just sugar!
- **Soybean Oil:** Genetically modified oil that's been refined
- **Xanthan Gum, Artificial Color, Phosphoric Acid, Polysorbate 60:** Definitely not real food items—plus one tells you directly it's fake!
- **Yellow 6, Yellow 5:** Chemical colorants
- **Natural Flavor:** This is often a pseudonym for chemicals or MSG.

Spaghetti Sauce

INGREDIENTS: TOMATOES, WATER, TOMATO CONCENTRATE, ONIONS, GARLIC, BASIL, SEA SALT, EXTRA VIRGIN OLIVE OIL, OREGANO, CITRIC ACID.

- This spaghetti sauce is full of real natural foods (citric acid is a natural acid found in fruits such as lemons and limes).
Great choice!

Menu Planning

To save time, plan your menu for the week ahead. If that seems overwhelming, start by tackling dinner plans first. Plan for a variety of proteins such as chicken, fish, beef, and meatless main dishes as well. For example, if you will be home six nights and your family eats pretty much everything, start with what they love. How many chicken dishes? Soups? Casseroles? Turkey? Meatless? Then fill in with vegetables, salads, and side dishes.

Then write up your menu to remind yourself what you will be cooking, and post it in the kitchen. This might even be a way to get the family involved in helping.

Master Grocery List

After you have planned your menu, create a master shopping list. Categorize items into the section of the grocery store such as produce, dairy, poultry and meat, frozen. Note what you have stocked in your pantry (dry or freezer) so you do not duplicate purchases or waste time. Buy most of what you need at once to save time, then pick up perishable items as needed throughout the week.

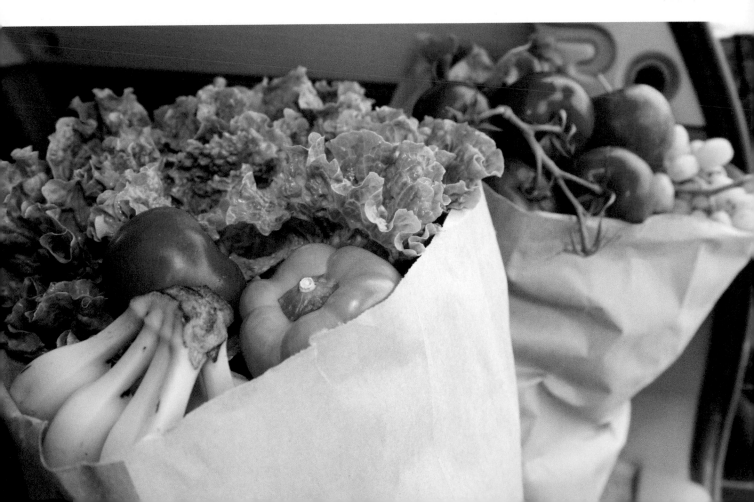

Food 101: Making the Best Choices

Vegetables and Fruits

As you shop for produce, gather lots of color. Focus on whole, fresh fruits and vegetables. Think about shopping the rainbow: The more color in your basket, the wider variety of flavors and textures you will taste and the broader range of nutrients you will be feeding your body. Be brave. Try new fruits and vegetables you are unfamiliar with. If you are not sure what something is, ask an employee in the produce section or at the farmers market table.

If you think you don't like a vegetable, think about why. Is it how it has been prepared? Is it the texture or seasoning? You can change that and maybe turn something previously disliked into a new favorite. Experiment!

Fresh vegetables not looking good or out of season? Check the frozen foods section. Many vegetables are harvested at their peak of flavor and nutrition and then flash-frozen to preserve the vitamins and minerals.

Daniel Plan cooking focuses on non-starchy vegetables and low-sugar (low-glycemic) fruits.

Health Benefits

Focusing on a diet filled with fruits and vegetables has been proven to improve health and fight lifestyle-related diseases such as diabetes, obesity, and heart disease. Moreover, a high consumption of fruits and vegetables has been shown to lower blood pressure, reduce the risk for stroke, and also reduce the risk of some cancers. It is even more important if you are a cancer survivor. As the Greek physician Hippocrates famously said more than two thousand years ago, food is definitely medicine.

Colleen Doyle, MS, RD, the nutrition director of the American Cancer Society in Atlanta, Georgia, says, "Our most important strategy for cancer prevention is improving the diet largely through fruit and vegetable consumption."

Nonstarchy Vegetables

Artichokes	Asparagus	Bell peppers	Broccoli
Broccolini	Brussels sprouts	Cabbage	Cauliflower
Celery	Cucumbers	Eggplant	Fennel
Green beans	Kale	Leeks	Mushrooms
Onions	Salad greens	Snap peas	Spinach
Summer squash	Swiss chard	Tomatoes	Zucchini

Low-sugar Fruits

Apples	Avocados	Apricots	Blackberries
Blueberries	Goji berries	Grapefruit	Kiwi
Nectarines	Peaches	Raspberries	

So you might be asking, where are my potatoes, peas, corn, and carrots? Aren't they good for me too? The answer is yes, they are good for you, but they are starchy vegetables. They are digested and stored as energy in your cells, but too much can contribute to high blood sugar levels. Think of them as a side dish in place of grains. Other familiar starchy veggies include parsnips, winter squash, pumpkins, sweet potatoes, yams, and rutabagas.

Check The Daniel Plan website (*daniel plan.com*) for a full list of recommended fruits and vegetables.

Lean Protein

Protein is a critical building block for our body. Protein builds and repairs tissues, and it makes enzymes, hormones, and other body chemicals. It is an important building block of bones, muscles, cartilage, skin, and blood. So what are the best sources of healthy protein?

Lean protein comes in both animal and plant options. Daniel Plan animal proteins include lean chicken, turkey, beef, and low-mercury sustainably caught seafood. Plant sources of protein include beans, seeds, peas, lentils, and nuts.

Animal Protein

When you shop, choose hormone-free poultry, low-mercury seafood, and grass-fed beef if possible, depending on availability and budget.

Think about portions when you are shopping. Generally 4–6 ounces of protein is plenty per serving. One pound to a pound and a half is all you need for four people. At the seafood counter, don't settle for a piece of fish that is too large. Ask them to cut what you want, and have them remove the skin for you. It saves time in the kitchen.

Poultry

Don't be fooled by a label claiming "all natural." It's meaningless. For options on buying high-quality poultry, check out *LocalHarvest.org*, where you can search for local poultry farmers who don't use antibiotics or arsenic in feed. Find farmers markets, family farms, and other sources of organic and sustainably grown food in your area.

If you can afford it, organic poultry ensures that what you are buying was raised without antibiotics, arsenic, hormones, and many other unappetizing drugs prevalent in conventionally grown poultry.

Beef

Look for grass-fed and pastured beef. Choose beef raised without unnecessary hormones and antibiotics. Talk with your butcher about the meat he sells. Ask questions. The most natural diet for cattle is grass, not corn.

Grass-fed beef is a leaner choice than corn-fed or finished beef and has a more favorable ratio of omega fatty acids. For helpful information on decoding grocery store labels and more about antibiotics, check out The Meat Eaters Guide from *EWG.org*.

The Dirty Dozen and Clean Fifteen Fruits and Vegetables

Each year the Environmental Working Group publishes a list called "The Dirty Dozen and The Clean Fifteen." The Dirty Dozen list will help you choose what fruits and vegetables are most important to buy organic to avoid high pesticide loads. The Clean Fifteen list will help you choose what is safe to buy conventionally grown.

When you shop, carry the "Shoppers Guide to Pesticides" from the Environmental Working Group (EWG). You can print it off of their website at *EWG.org*.

If your grocery budget is tight, this information will help you make wise choices and maximize your shopping dollars.

Seafood

Fish is a rich source of omega-3 fats, which help to improve cardiovascular health, boost the immune system, lower the risk for heart disease, and lower inflammation, which contributes to many chronic illnesses. Unfortunately, many fish are high in mercury. So choose wild and sustainably caught seafood as much as possible. Choose low-mercury salmon, mackerel, trout, sardines, tuna, halibut, and other options. Download the pocket seafood guide from *SeafoodWatch.org* for current information on the best seafood choices and good alternatives.

Plant Protein

Beans (dried and canned), seeds (think flax, quinoa, hemp, millet), legumes, lentils, and nuts are great sources of healthy, plant-based protein. They also add fiber, vitamins, and minerals to your body. Nuts also add a good dose of healthy fat. If your grocery budget is tight, increasing plant-based protein is an economical option.

Beans

Whether dried or canned, beans are a versatile ingredient and pantry staple. Beans are also a superfood—a food that is nutrient-dense and packed with nutrition. In addition to protein, beans add calcium, iron, potassium, and B vitamins. Beans can be made into soups, stews, and dips; tossed into salads; and added to grains and pastas. Beans can be the star of a dish or a supporting player.

When shopping for dried beans, buy from a store that has good turnover and use dried beans within a year of purchase. When buying canned beans, look for BPA-free cans. BPA (Bisphenol-A) is an industrial chemical that leaches into food and drink from cans and polycarbonate plastics.

Another bean listed on The Daniel Plan is the soybean, or edamame. Although soy is controversial and an ingredient in many highly processed foods, whole soybeans can be a healthy option. Soybeans are an excellent source of plant protein. Be sure to choose organic soybeans, since conventionally grown soybeans will be from genetically modified crops. Find shelled organic edamame in the frozen food aisle. Add them to rice dishes, pasta, quinoa, and salads.

Seeds (Pseudo-Grains)

If you are new to seed grains, you may think you are looking at birdseed! When we say seeds, we are talking about ingredients often treated as grains, such as quinoa, teff, millet, amaranth, hemp seed, chia seed, and buckwheat. These are seed grains in contrast to cereal grains.

Many seeds are complete proteins. A complete protein has all twenty amino acids. Our bodies use amino acids to form thousands of proteins our bodies need to function. Our bodies can make eleven amino acids; we must get the other nine from our diet.

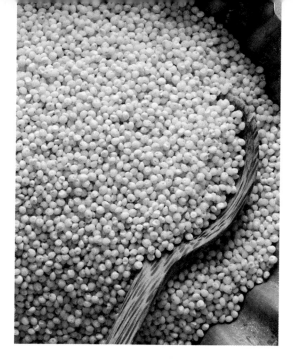

Grain and Flours

When enjoyed in controlled quantities, grains can add healthy, plant-based protein to our diet. A good source of complex carbohydrates, grains also add important vitamins, minerals, and fiber.

Whole Grains Defined

Let's start with a definition to clarify things. There are whole grains and refined grains. The Daniel Plan focus is on healthy whole grains—grains that have not been stripped of their bran (the tough outer layer) and germ (rich in vitamins, minerals, and unsaturated oils). Processing strips away much of the vitamins and fiber.

Seed grains are easy to cook and hold well refrigerated for the better part of a week. Make a big batch to use in a variety of ways. They can be enjoyed for breakfast, as salads for lunch or snacks, as side dishes for dinner, and in soups and stews.

Whole grains are better sources of fiber and contain key vitamins and minerals. Better yet, eating whole grains has been linked to a lower risk of heart disease, diabetes, some cancers, and other health problems.

Food Sensitivities

There is a lot of controversy, superstition, and confusion surrounding the subject of food allergies, sensitivities, and illness. To clear up the confusion, we want to tell you that the two most common foods that trigger reactions are gluten (found in wheat, barley, rye, and spelt) and dairy. These foods activate inflammation, which is the root of autoimmune diseases. The rise of these food sensitivities now is directly related to what we have been eating. Our processed, low-fiber, high-sugar diet alters the bacteria that live in our digestive system. So if you have chronic health concerns, we encourage you to eliminate gluten and dairy from your diet for a minimum of ten days to see if you are sensitive to these foods. We encourage you to check out our DP detox in *The Daniel Plan* or try some of the dozens of gluten-free and dairy-free options and recipes in this book.

In the whole grains category (sometimes called cereal grains), healthy options include rice (brown, red, purple, black, and wild), barley, rye, faro, bulgur, kamut, oats (rolled or steel cut), corn, spelt, and whole wheat. This includes pastas such as brown rice, whole grain, and multi-grain.

Flours

Most whole grains are also available ground into flour. You will find whole wheat flour, rice flour, corn flour, corn polenta, and seed grain flours such as quinoa, teff, buckwheat, and many more. Look for producers such as Bob's Red Mill, King Arthur, and Arrowhead Mills at markets across the country and online. These makers also produce gluten-free flour blends that can be used just like regular flour. Gluten-free flours are usually based on rice flours, tapioca, cornstarch, bean flours, sorghum, and potato starch. Each maker has its own special blend, or you can buy the flours individually and blend your own.

Unfortunately, while they sound healthy, many whole wheat flours are almost as refined as white flours. Whole wheat flours should be unbleached and unrefined.

Another "flour" you will find are nut flours, also called "meals." They are made from very finely ground nuts. Often used for baking and in place of or in combination with bread crumbs, nut flours add a nice nutty flavor and color. Nut flours work in both sweet and savory recipes and are gluten-free.

When storing whole grain, seed, and nut flours, you should place many in the refrigerator or freezer to preserve freshness because of higher oil content. Check the label to see what the manufacturer recommends.

Breads, Crackers, and Wraps

There is debate over whether breads, crackers, and wraps are processed foods. Some are; some are not. Reading labels will help you make a wise choice. Is it bread or

Whole Wheat — Is It Real?

So is it really a whole grain, or is it refined white flour with caramel coloring masquerading as a whole grain?

When shopping, you may see a familiar yellow stamp from the Whole Grains Council. Their label lets you know that one serving of this product contains at least 8 grams of a whole grain, or half a serving. However, if the label says whole grain, it does not mean it is 100 percent whole grain. It could be only 51 percent whole grain by weight and the rest refined grains, sugar, and sodium.

Look for unbleached whole grain wheat or 100 percent whole wheat in the ingredient list. A whole grain product should list an actual whole grain as its first ingredient.

a cracker that you could have made your-self, with simple real ingredients? Beware of sugar, sodium, partially hydrogenated oils (dangerous fats), "natural" ingredients, artificial coloring, artificial flavoring, and ingredients you cannot pronounce.

For wraps, look for organic corn tortillas (sprouted grain if you can get them), 100 percent whole wheat or multi-grain torti-llas, and brown rice tortillas. Check out the refrigerated section for options, not just end caps and bread aisles. For gluten-free wraps, choose corn or choose blends made with teff, millet, other gluten-free grains, or coconut.

Fiber

An essential part of everyone's diet, fiber is the part of plants that our bodies cannot digest or absorb. Dietary fiber is what your mom might have politely called *roughage*. Fiber helps us feel full, keeps things mov-ing with digestion, balances blood sugar, and aids us in achieving and maintaining a healthy weight. A high-fiber diet also helps prevent diseases such as diabetes, heart disease, obesity, and digestive problems.

Fiber comes in two forms: soluble and insoluble. Soluble fiber dissolves in water and forms a gel-like substance that moves food through the digestive system. Insoluble fiber does not dissolve in water and rapidly passes through the digestive system.

If, like most people, your diet is lacking the 25–40 grams of recommended fiber

per day, The Daniel Plan food principles will improve that. But you can also up your fiber by increasing your consump-tion of flax seeds or chia seeds. Add them to a bowl of oatmeal or buckwheat or to smoothies, or salads.

Eggs and Dairy

Eggs got a bad report card years ago, but their reputation has been restored. And to retire another myth, eggs do not raise your cholesterol. Eggs are a healthy form of protein.

When you are buying eggs, sev-eral options will help you find the best: organic, free-range, cage-free, pastured, or omega-3 eggs. Eggs enhanced or enriched by omega-3 come from chickens whose feed is supplemented with an omega-3 source such as flax seeds.

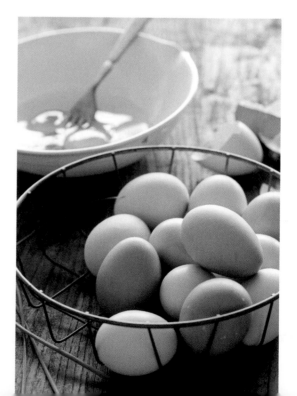

Although famous faces sport milk mustaches in glossy magazines and on billboards, we don't need to drink milk to be healthy. Of the world's population, 75 percent are lactose intolerant. Lactose-intolerant people cannot digest the natural sugar in milk.

You will find that we use milk alternatives in a number of Daniel Plan recipes. Many people who have trouble digesting cow's milk do better with goat or sheep milks and cheeses. Those make excellent substitutes.

Enjoy dairy in moderation if it agrees with you. Choose organic, pasture-raised products when possible, and try full-fat versus low-fat dairy products. This might surprise you. Full fat? Yes, it is more satisfying; therefore, you will likely eat less.

Cheese

In this cookbook a few recipes use cheese in moderation. Generally, go for hard or firm cheeses, not processed cheese. Full-fat cheese will give you more satisfaction. And big flavor cheeses, such as Parmesan-Reggiano or extra-sharp cheddar, add so much flavor that just a little is all you need.

Be smart about portion control. An ounce of a hard cheese is approximately 1-inch square. If organic is not available, choose a brand that does not use artificial growth hormones. The label should read without rBGH or rBST.

A dairy-free option for cheese replacement is nutritional yeast, because of its cheese-like taste. Nutritional yeast is inactive yeast with no fermenting power. It is a good source of protein, dietary fiber, vitamins, and minerals. It is also sodium-free and gluten-free. Nutritional yeast is available in most markets in the healthy food aisle.

Yogurt

Fermented dairy such as yogurt and kefir contain beneficial bacteria that are good

Dairy Alternatives

There are many alternatives to cow's milk for smoothies and general cooking needs such as sheep's or goat's milk and "milks" made from almonds, cashews, rice, oats, hemp, coconut, and soy. They come packed in shelf-stable boxes and in the refrigerated dairy section.

Almond milk is popular and easy to make at home with raw almonds (see page 80). Unfortunately, some boxed brands add ingredients such as sugar and carrageenan, a "natural" food additive that can cause digestive issues and inflammation for some people. While boxed versions are convenient, they may not be the best choice.

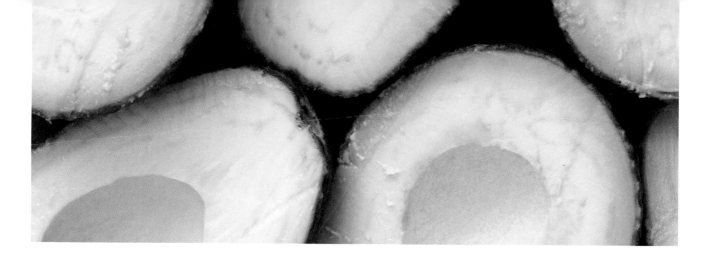

for our digestive systems. Greek-style yogurt has skyrocketed in popularity. With its thick, rich texture and tangy taste, it's easy to understand why. Greek yogurt is thicker because of a straining process. Straining gives it that creamy texture while removing liquid whey and some lactose (natural milk sugar), making it less likely to upset lactose-intolerant people.

Because it takes two-to–four times more milk to make Greek-style yogurt, it has higher protein content than regular yogurt. Buy only plain, unsweetened Greek yogurt without thickeners or stabilizers. (As with all dairy, choose organic if you can.) Flavored varieties have a lot of added sugar. If you want a little sweetness, add a teaspoon of honey, maple syrup, or molasses. Or try adding a handful of fresh or frozen unsweetened berries.

Superfoods

While there is no official or medical definition, superfoods are foods that provide concentrated nutrients. Think of them as nutritional powerhouses. Superfoods deliver by leaps and bounds beyond basic nutrition in terms of vitamins, minerals, antioxidants, and phytonutrients (plant nutrients) for stellar health benefits. You might be eating superfoods already without knowing it.

Most whole foods that have intense colors are superfoods, such as avocados, blueberries, blackberries, tomatoes, broccoli, kale, yams and sweet potatoes, salmon, tomatoes, nuts, beans, seeds, and many others. The benefits of eating superfoods could fill an entire book!

Superfoods contribute to reducing inflammation, regulating metabolism, and lowering cholesterol and blood pressure; protect against heart disease and some cancers; and promote digestive health. They also have bold, tasty flavors. What more reasons could we ask for to add superfoods to our diet!

For optimum health, incorporate more superfoods (many are available in powder or seed form) into your daily diet. Here is a list to get you started:

Superfood	Benefits	Uses
Acai	Loaded with antioxidants, which help prevent diseases such as cancer, heart disease, stroke, Alzheimer's, rheumatoid arthritis, and cataracts	Add to smoothies and plain yogurt. Look for frozen acai puree (without added sugar) and freeze-dried acai powder.
Avocado	Anti-inflammatory, fiber-rich, high in folate, vitamins E and K, potassium and magnesium; provides heart-healthy fat	Add them to salads, wraps, omelets, sandwiches, dips, burgers, tacos, guacamole, or eat them all by themselves.
Beans	Inexpensive source of protein, calcium, iron, potassium, vitamin B, manganese, magnesium, fiber; support healthy blood sugar	Make soups and stews with beans; add to salads, chilis, and dips. Beans are versatile and hearty.
Berries (blackberries, raspberries, blueberries, strawberries)	Offer disease-fighting antioxidants and anthocyanins, vitamin C, potassium, memory support, fiber; reduce cancer risk; are anti-inflammatory	Add berries to smoothies or cereals; enjoy as a snack or dessert; add to green salads, plain Greek yogurt, or as part of a fruit salad.
Broccoli/ Broccolini	Anti-inflammatory, detoxifying, and cancer-fighting; contains antioxidants, vitamin C, vitamin E, manganese, zinc and high fiber	Enjoy warm or chilled as a side dressed with a lemony vinaigrette or a drizzle of good olive oil. Throw into a soup, or eat raw with a dip.
Cacao (raw)	Has antioxidants and essential minerals, including iron, zinc, copper, calcium, magnesium, and fiber; builds strong bones, promotes cardiovascular health, decreases depression, lifts mood, promotes relaxation, and decreases blood pressure	Add to a smoothie for breakfast, use in desserts, or mix into plain Greek yogurt with a little stevia.
Chia	Source of omega-3 fats, protein, vitamins, minerals, antioxidants, and fiber	Chia seeds have a neutral flavor and the ability to absorb liquids and work as a thickener. Sprinkle in oatmeal, smoothies, and dips. Try them in a lentil stew or soup.
Coconut water	Is high in key electrolytes sodium, magnesium, calcium, potassium, and phosphorus; supports hydration and provides minerals such as manganese and iron	As a great rehydrator after exercise, use in smoothies. Look for the organic, freeze-dried powder you can carry and mix with water or tea. Mix it into breakfast porridge.

Superfood	Benefits	Uses
Flax seed	Offers heart-healthy omega-3 fats, fiber and lignans, which are high in antioxidants.	Add to smoothies, cereals, yogurt, burgers, and salads. Flax mixed with water can be used as an egg substitute for vegans in some recipes. Mix into baked goods such as pizza crusts, muffins, waffles, pancakes.
Garlic	Provides anti-cancer, anti-viral, antioxidant, and anti- inflammatory benefits; promotes cardiovascular health	Garlic provides wonderful flavor to soups, stews, flavor dressings, side dishes, and just about every savory dish you can think of. Cooking and roasting mellow its pungent raw flavor, making it almost sweet.
Green and black tea	Rich in lycopene and flavonoids, powerful, protective, and plant-based compounds that promote health, help the body get rid of toxins, are anti-inflammatory, and reduce risk of cancer, heart disease, Alzheimer's, and dementia	Enjoy iced or warm any time of the day and iced after a workout to replenish fluids.
Grapefruit	An excellent source of antioxidant vitamin C, anti-inflammatory, and for lowering bad cholesterol; also, lycopene in pink and red grapefruit	Eat for breakfast, add segments to green salads, or make a fruit salad.

Note: If you take statin drugs, check with your doctor before eating grapefruit.

Superfood	Benefits	Uses
Hemp	A complete protein, providing all essential amino acids; also providing minerals, including magnesium, iron, zinc, and potassium	Add to smoothies, salads, and oatmeal; sprinkle over berries and Greek yogurt; or make hemp milk. Use it as a protein powder. Available in both seed and powder form.
Kale	Provides high levels of vitamins A, C, and K; phytonutrients; and minerals copper, potassium, iron, manganese, and phosphorus and fiber; loaded with antioxidants and promoting eye health	Make a salad, cook as a side vegetable, use in a green smoothie.

Note: Anyone taking anticoagulant meds should check with a doctor before eating kale or any vegetable high in vitamin K.

Superfood	Benefits	Uses
Oats	High in fiber and rich in magnesium, potassium, zinc, copper, manganese, selenium, thiamine, and pantothenic acid; provides powerful phytonutrients	Good for breakfast. Add other superfoods to the bowl, such as hemp seeds, chia seeds, and berries.
Onions	Offers many healthy benefits from compounds called fructans, flavonoids, and organosulfur (that make eyes tear when we cut them); cancer-fighters and bone-strengtheners; allergy relievers	They go into just about everything: soups, stews, and all savory dishes. Grill them for burgers, and chop into salads. Shallots have the same benefits.
Pomegranate	Pack a punch of flavonoids and polyphenols, potent antioxidants in the fight against cancer and heart disease	Sprinkle seeds in a green salad, over Greek yogurt, along with other berries; add to buckwheat or oatmeal; add to a fruit salad; stir into cooked rice; garnish soup or chicken as a tart balance to a savory dish.
Pumpkin	High-fiber fruit (not vegetable) providing loads of vitamin C and E and disease-fighting nutrients in the rich orange flesh, plus potassium, magnesium, and pantothenic acid; good for hearts, eyes, skin, and bones	Make soup or stew; add a swirl to plain yogurt with a few drops of stevia and a sprinkle of nuts for breakfast or a snack. It's available fresh in season and available year-round canned.
Quinoa	A complete protein that provides all essential amino acids	Enjoy warm or cold as a salad or side dish; warm for a breakfast porridge; combine with vegetables for a quick lunch. Keep a container of cooked quinoa in the fridge at all times, ready to go.
Salmon (wild)	High levels of healthy omega-3 fats and selenium; anti-inflammatory; promotes better brain function, decreased risk of cardiovascular problems, cancer, and eye health benefits	Sear, roast, grill, or poach for lunch or dinner; add to salads. Make salmon chowder, burgers, or cakes. Canned salmon can make a good snack.
Sweet potatoes	A good source of vitamins A and C, manganese, and potassium; high level of the antioxidant beta-carotene; helps lower the risk posed by heavy metals and benefits those with digestive problems; anti-inflammatory; blood sugar regulation properties	Whip, roast, steam, or bake them into healthy "fries." Try a sprinkle of chopped walnuts. Add warm spices for extra flavor. They are even good cold-packed for lunch away from home.

Superfood	Benefits	Uses
Tomatoes	Rich in antioxidants, vitamins C, A, and K, and beta-carotene; reduce the risk for heart disease and cancer	Toss into salads, use in wraps, pizzas, sandwiches, make marinara and soup, add to chili — you can do so many things with tomatoes! Choose organic.
Walnuts	Help the heart and circulatory system, offer cancer-fighting benefits, and support blood sugar control; anti-inflammatory; support bone health	Add flavor and crunch by sprinkling on salads, enjoy as a snack, add to breakfast oatmeal or porridge, add to vegetables and just about anything.

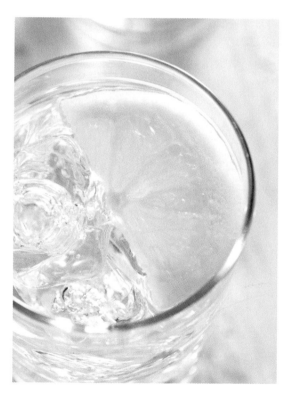

The Wonders of Water: Staying Hydrated

Good, clean, simple, pure water. Water is life. It is amazing stuff, and we often take it for granted. Because our bodies are 55 to 75 percent water, staying hydrated is critical to being healthy. Every part of our bodies needs hydration to function properly.

Water helps regulate our blood pressure and body temperature, improves circulation, and impacts our heart rate. Water raises our metabolism, helps us to feel full, removes wastes, lubricates joints, and boosts energy. Water helps prevent muscle cramping, flushes out impurities, and gives our skin a glow.

When we don't get enough water, we may feel hungry, tired, and mentally foggy or get a headache. For athletes, poor hydration might result in poor performance.

Healthy Hydrators

While fruits and vegetables have high water content and contribute to our overall hydration level, we also need to consume plenty of liquids. Sodas, coffee drinks, sugary drinks, sweetened ice tea, and neon sports drinks do not qualify.

If you like the fizz of soda, try sparkling water or mineral water. For flavor, add a squeeze of lemon, lime, or orange, or all three. Add a little natural juice such as pomegranate or watermelon juice (puree watermelon chunks in the blender and strain) mixed with lime. Add fresh mint leaves or a cucumber slice for a refreshing option. For a little sweetness, try a few drops of liquid stevia, or stir in a little whole leaf stevia powder.

Coconut water is an excellent hydrator. As the clear liquid center that is tapped from young, green coconuts, coconut water is a naturally great hydrator. (Just be sure to read labels for any added sugar.) Coconut water contains electrolytes, which are often lost during exercise or illness. You can even get powdered organic coconut, which is easily transportable. Add to water for an instant hydrator or to a morning smoothie.

Hydrated or Dehydrated: The Signals

How can you tell if your body is hydrated? If urine is light colored or clear, you are hydrated. If it is dark yellow, you need water. And if you are thirsty or have a dry mouth, your body is signaling that you are more dehydrated than you realize.

How much you need varies with hot weather (and how much we sweat), altitude, general health (more during illness or pregnancy), activity level, age (kids and men needing more than women), medications, gender, and body size. A good starting point is to aim for half of your body weight in fluid ounces and go from there. Listen to your body: If you are thirsty, you are already dehydrated.

Depending on where you live, tap water may not be as safe and clean as you might

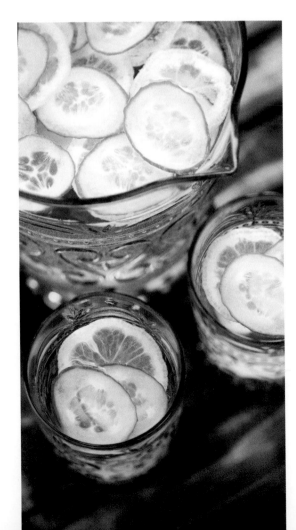

think. It's wise to use some sort of water filter to have access to fresh, pure water.

Skip the cost of bottled water and buy refillable, BPA-free plastic or stainless steel bottles. Wash them daily. Carry water everywhere, and you will remember to drink it throughout the day.

Sugar and Sweeteners

We probably do not have to tell you how bad sugar is for you. If you are eating whole, fresh healthy foods; skipping fast, junk, and processed foods; and don't drink soda or sugary drinks, you have already done a good job eliminating a lot of sugar.

We must be highly aware of how much sugar we consume and then work to minimize it in our diets. We are talking mostly about added sugars and hidden sugars—for which there are over 250 names on ingredient labels! If an ingredient ends in -ose, it is sugar.

Also be cautious of falling into the artificial sweeteners trap. Beware of aspartame, acesulfame, and anything that ends in -ol, such as maltitol, sorbitol, and xylitol.

They are used in foods labeled sugar-free. These substitutes are sugar alcohols, a sort of hybrid carb between sugar and alcohol. Our bodies have a hard time breaking them down, and they can cause digestive problems.

What about agave and stevia? While marketed as a healthy alternative, agave is controversial because most brands are high in fructose. One brand that is low in fructose (at 47 percent, considered low on the glycemic index) is Xagave. Since agave is sweeter than sugar, you can use less.

So what about that occasional sweet tooth or treat? The good news is, it is okay to tolerate a little sugar on occasion. Skip refined sugar, which has no value. Try a little natural sweetener, such as raw honey, pure maple syrup, molasses, or organic sucanat—a whole unrefined cane sugar.

If a sweet attack comes, try enjoying a piece of naturally fresh fruit, berries, an ounce of 70 percent bittersweet chocolate, or even sweet vegetables such as yams. Once you get rid of refined and artificial sugars, your taste buds will adjust and you won't crave these kinds of foods.

Stevia

Stevia is an all-natural sweetener that comes from a plant—and the bonus is that it has no calories. When buying stevia, choose the original, whole-plant extract, in liquid or powder form that has no additives and is not mixed with artificial sweeteners.

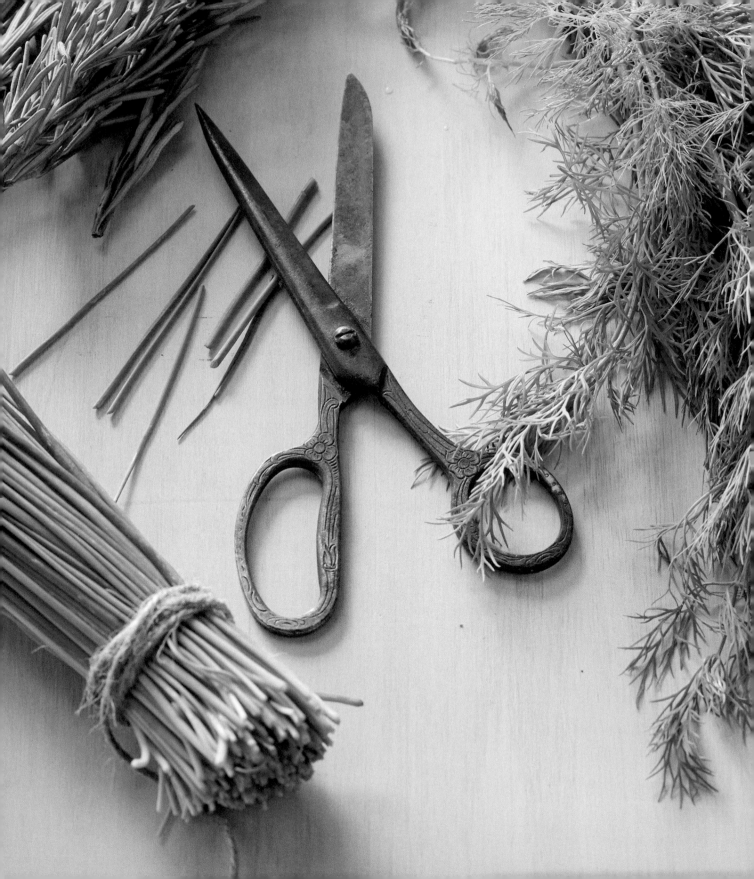

Basic Cooking Essentials

Herbs and Spices

Reading The Daniel Plan recipes, you will see that we use lots of herbs and spices to add flavor. We couldn't live without them! Spices are aromatic seasonings that usually come from seeds, buds, fruit, berries, and the bark or roots of plants and trees. Think of cinnamon, pepper, cloves, ginger, cumin, and coriander.

While you can grow fresh herbs in spring and summer, in colder months you have two options: buy fresh packages from the grocery store, or use dried herbs. Most stores sell fresh herbs year round in the produce department. Herbs and spices not only add flavor, texture, and color to food, but are also good for you. Many have anti-inflammatory, immune system–boosting, and antioxidant properties.

One thing we use a lot of that is thought of as an herb or spice, but is neither, is garlic. Related to leeks and onions, garlic is actually a vegetable and offers tremendous health benefits.

A few tips on cooking with herbs and spices:

- Use three times as many fresh herbs as dried. Dried herbs have more concentrated flavor; 1 tablespoon fresh = 1 teaspoon dried.

- Dried herbs need time to rehydrate in a recipe, so they are best with longer cooking times, about an hour, as in soups, stews, and some sauces.

- Add fresh herbs toward the end of cooking or as garnish for extra flavor.

- Dried herbs last about 6–12 months before losing their potency. Spices last about 1 year. Whole spices (whole nutmeg, peppercorns, coriander seed) will last longer.

- For the freshest spices, use a small, inexpensive coffee grinder to grind whole spices. Keep it just for spices, and not for coffee.

- Date a bottle each time you open one.

- Buy herbs and spices in small quantities unless you use a lot of one in particular; then a large size will save money.

Herb/Spice	Benefits
Cinnamon	Can lower blood sugar and support good cholesterol—sprinkle some in your morning smoothie, oatmeal, or pancake batter.
Turmeric	Contains curcumin, a powerful anti-inflammatory—add some to rice or soups.
Paprika, chili powders, cayenne	Contain capsaicin, which gives these spices their heat (in varying levels). Capsaicin is anti-inflammatory and has been associated with pain relief, unless you eat too much of the hot stuff.
Oregano	Has anti-bacterial, antioxidant, anti-viral, and disease-fighting properties; also high in iron and manganese. Oregano is great with tomatoes, in sauces, and with eggs, grains, poultry, vegetables—almost anything.
Rosemary	Contains substances that boost the immune system, improve digestion, and act as an anti-inflammatory. Rosemary is a classic match with chicken.
Cilantro	Is a known detoxifier with high levels of antioxidants and acts as a digestive aid. Add to Mexican dishes for a fresh note.

- Store herbs and spices in a cool, dark place in your pantry or in a drawer, not near or above the stove, where it is hot and humid.

- Using herbs and spices to lift food flavors is a good way to reduce sodium in your diet.

- Salt and pepper are foundational in cooking and for seasoning your food. Use salt sensibly; Kosher and sea salts pack more impact, so you won't use as much. Or try artisanal salts and peppers.

Fats

Let's get one thing out of the way. Fat is not the enemy. While eating low-fat was the mantra of healthy-eating proponents for many years, the message missed the mark. Fat is an essential part of our diets, but it must be healthy fat—and the right amount.

Fat satisfies us, transports flavor, balances our blood sugar, settles our hunger, and helps us use the fat-soluble vitamins our bodies require to function: A, D, E, and K. But not all fats are created equal.

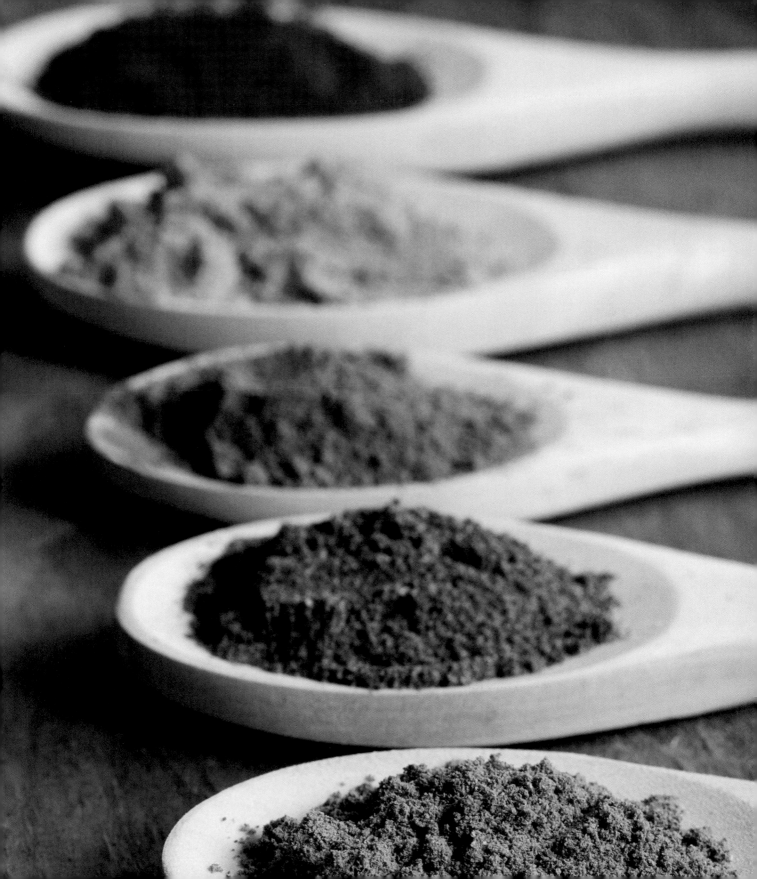

Here are tips to keep your body running like a well-oiled machine.

The Good Fats

The good fats are known as monoun-saturated (MUFAs) and polyunsaturated (PUFAs). Both help to reduce the risk for heart disease and stroke, reduce blood pressure, and improve cholesterol. These healthy fats are also usually high in Vitamin E, something many people need more of. But they are still fats and high in calories, so enjoy in moderation.

Good sources of healthy fats include:

- Avocados
- Nuts
- Nut butters
- Olives
- Fish
- Seeds
- Oils

Choosing Oils

If you have the standard jug of "vegetable" oil lurking in your pantry, toss it. It is most likely soybean, corn, or canola oil, pro-cessed at high heat with toxic solvents and chemicals (such as hexane).

The better choice? Healthy oils labeled cold-pressed or expeller-pressed. Pressing or grinding seeds or fruit mechanically with heavy granite millstones or stainless steel presses at low heat produces these oils. They are not produced with high heat or industrial chemicals. Oils produced this way retain their flavor and, more importantly, their nutrition and health benefits. These healthy fats are typically liquid at room temperature, compared with solids such as shortening, margarine, or butter.

For healthy cooking, we recommend unrefined extra-virgin olive oil, coconut oil (firm at cooler room temperatures), grape seed oil, avocado oil, and sesame oil.

Tips on Oils

Choose unrefined oils as much as pos-sible. These oils are closest to their natural state, with all health benefits intact. Pass on mass-market, lower-quality oils. They are often refined to mask poor quality or impurities.

Storage: Many oils come in dark green bottles or metal cans to protect them from light, which is good. Light and heat cause oils to go rancid more quickly. If oil is in a clear glass bottle, store it in a cool, dark place such as your pantry to protect it and extend the shelf life. Coconut oil is an exception. It generally comes in clear jars without risk. As it warms up, it quickly liq-uefies. Some oils, like sesame and other nut oils, are better stored in the refrigerator to preserve their quality, flavor, and longevity.

Most oils will last about six months after opening. Be sure to check for any "use by" dates on the labels before you buy.

Smoke point: Cooking oils have differ-ent "smoke points," or temperatures where they start to smoke and break down. If you accidently turn your back on a pan with

Oil	The Skinny	Cooking Temperature
Extra-virgin olive oil	With a wide range of flavors from fruity, grassy, and peppery and mild to strong, extra-virgin olive oil is one of the most widely loved heart-healthy oils in the world. It also can be found in many price ranges from everyday cooking oils to finishing oils. Find a mild, fruity, moderately priced oil for everyday use. The more expensive estate or reserve olive oil or oils from a single varietal such as Arbequina are best used as finishing oils. They are usually produced in smaller quantities, as they have unique and delicate flavors that heat might damage. Use them to drizzle over salad greens, cooked fish, chicken, and vegetables. Think of them as a sauce. Even a few drops can provide amazing flavor.	Good for up to medium temperatures
Coconut oil	Cast as a villain in the past because it is a saturated fat, coconut oil has been shown to be a health hero and smart choice. It has been enjoyed by tropical cultures for thousands of years. Coconut oil contains an anti-inflammatory fat called lauric acid; offers anti-bacterial, anti-fungal, and anti-viral benefits; and supports blood sugar control and good cholesterol. Unrefined oil has a definite coconut flavor. Some brands have more or less flavor than others. Experiment and find a brand you enjoy the taste of. It is solid at room temperature and liquefies around 77 degrees. Coconut oil is good for cooking chicken, fish, and vegetables, where the unique flavor of coconut complements the overall flavor of the dish. It can add an Asian or tropical flair. Choose a brand that has not been bleached or deodorized.	Good for up to medium-high temperatures
Grape seed oil	A by-product of winemaking, grape seed oil has a clean, light flavor making it the perfect alternative to vegetable oil. Its neutral flavor allows other flavors to shine, such as herbs and spices. It's also nice when you don't want to taste the flavor of the oil in your recipes. Grape seed oil is a good source of vitamin E and oleic acid, which may reduce the risk of stroke and reduce hunger pangs. It is also a rich source of linoleic acid, which fights heart disease and bad cholesterol.	Good for up to medium-high temperatures

(continued)

Oil	The Skinny	Cooking Temperature
Avocado oil	Avocado oil helps to improve cholesterol and has anti-inflammatory compounds. It also supplies lutein, an antioxidant important for eye health. Versatile avocado oil also has a very high smoke point, about 520°, making it the perfect choice for high-heat cooking needs such as grilling, pan-roasting, and sautéing. Its wonderful buttery flavor also makes delicious vinaigrettes and dressing for salads and vegetables.	Good general-purpose oil that can be used up to high temperatures
Sesame oil	Nice for stir-fries and lending an Asian flair to many dishes, unrefined sesame oil is highly fragrant and adds robust flavor. Try drizzling it over cooked or raw vegetables too. Just a few drops will do!	Good for up to medium-high temperatures
Nut oils, flaxseed oil	Save specialty oils such as these for using to dress salads and drizzle over vegetables, salads, seafood, and chicken. These oils are best not heated for cooking, as heat can destroy their delicate flavors and health benefits.	Do not cook

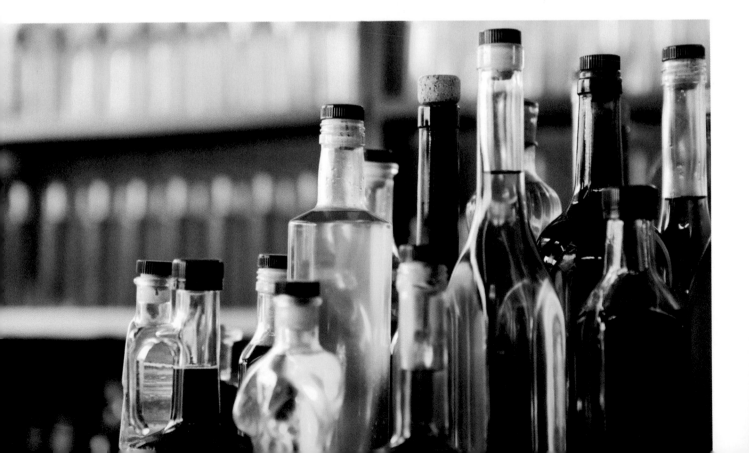

oil and it gets too hot and starts smoking? Allow it to cool a bit, wipe out with paper towels, and start over. Any smoking oil is unhealthy because it releases carcinogens into the air and damaging free radicals into the oil.

Good oil gone bad: If an oil ever smells odd, like diesel fuel, it is probably rancid or spoiled. Time to replace it.

Other Fats: Butter, Margarine, Spreads, and More

We have talked a lot about oils, so you might be asking, what about butter, margarine, or spreads?

Butter

While The Daniel Plan uses minimal dairy, a little organic butter from pastured, grass-fed cows won't kill you. Butter is a saturated fat, so enjoy it in a small amount on occasion.

Margarine, Buttery Spreads, and Alternatives

At one time, margarine was considered the healthy replacement for butter. Unfortunately, it is not. Because of how most margarine is produced, through hydrogenation (an industrial process), it contains trans fats. Trans fats are the most dangerous types of fats in our diets, the ones we need to eliminate. So skip hydrogenated and partially hydrogenated margarine (or any fats), and opt for natural, healthier fats.

The Daniel Plan does approve of using a spread such as Earth Balance Buttery Spread and Coconut Spread as healthy options. Look for products that are made with all natural expeller-pressed oils; made with no artificial preservatives, flavors, colors, or emulsifiers; and are not hydrogenated.

Condiments

Although we probably sound like a broken record at this point, we cannot emphasize how important it is to read labels. For yet another example, let's address America's favorite dressing and spread: mayonnaise.

While it is easy to blindly grab your old favorite off the grocery store shelf, check out brands that may be unfamiliar. There are brands that use wholesome and natural ingredients. They don't sound like a science project when you read the label. You will find them not only on the shelf, but also in the refrigerated section of your market.

There are brands made with or without eggs, with no preservatives, and using expeller-pressed oils. Several brands to look for, among others, are made by Follow Your Heart Foods (Vegenaise) and Spectrum Organics. Pass on brands with preservatives, hydrogenated oils, or unhealthy additives such as EDTA.

For condiments such as ketchup, mustard, hoisin, barbecue sauce, teriyaki sauce, and many others, follow the same guidelines. Generally, organic versions omit the additives and unhealthy ingredients.

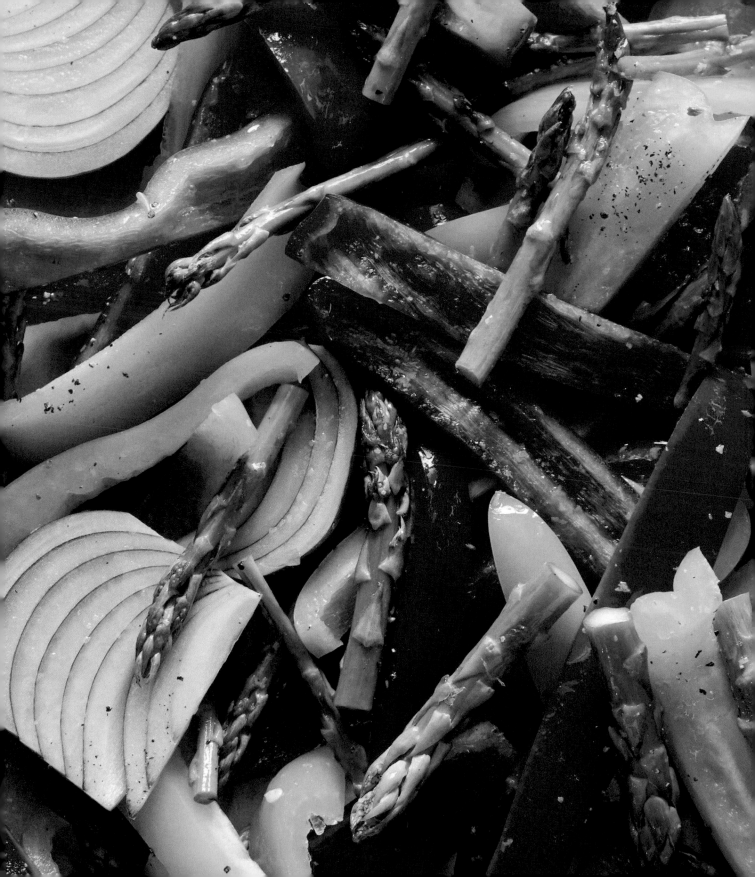

Tips and Guides

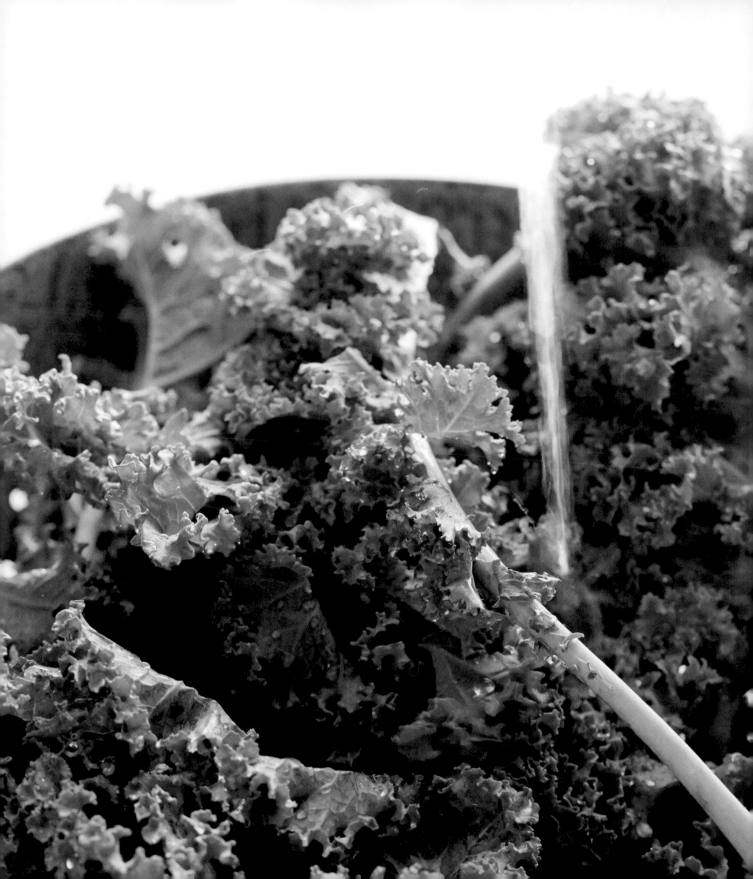

Time-Savers

1. Cook once; eat twice. Plan for leftovers you can use in a new way. *Leftovers* is not a dirty word! It's smart and efficient for a time-starved schedule. For example, roast extra chicken to use for chicken salad or chicken tacos. Make extra soup for lunch. That extra steak from the stir-fry? Add it to salad greens for a steak salad.

2. On busy nights, choose quick recipes such as boneless, skinless chicken breasts or baked seafood. Most of our recipes are designed to be quick and easy.

3. Make extra amounts of sauce recipes. Many freeze well and can be used in multiple ways to make new dishes during the week.

4. Gather dinner ingredients the night before or in the morning. Stack nonperishable ingredients on a rimmed baking sheet along with the recipe, so they are ready to go when you walk in the door.

5. Chop vegetables and measure them out ahead of time to save time when preparing a recipe, especially if the ingredient list has lots of vegetables. Just label and refrigerate until needed. When your ingredients are prepped ahead and ready (a French term called *mise en place*), recipes go more quickly. For quick salads, buy head lettuce, wash in cold water, spin dry in a salad spinner, and store in the refrigerator in a tight container.

6. Cook a few dishes or even meals ahead, package, and refrigerate. Most foods (except seafood) will last several days in the refrigerator. Just heat and enjoy.

7. Get the family involved and ask for help. Cooking is better together! In the kitchen everyone learns essential skills and healthy habits that will benefit them for a lifetime.

8. When you walk in the door, turn the oven on or get that pan of water boiling to save a few minutes.

9. With beans, soak overnight for cooking the next day. For canned beans, rinse, drain, and package for quick use.

Cost-Savers

1. Bulk purchasing will save you money. Be sure to shop from a store with good turnover of bulk grocery items.

2. Compare prices. Look at the unit price per item, such as cost per ounce, for better deals.

3. When cooking chicken, buy a whole bird and have the butcher cut it up or cut it up yourself. Whole chickens are usually less expensive than the pieces.

4. Use coupons if they match up with what you need to buy.

5. Buy in-season produce for best prices, especially foods such as berries for smoothies. Berries freeze easily.

6. Shop using the Dirty Dozen and Clean Fifteen lists to maximize your budget when buying organic.

7. Stock up, within reason, when often-used items are on sale such as canned beans, tomatoes, and broth.

8. Many things freeze well, so if it is on sale, buy extra and freeze. Just don't let it get lost and forgotten in the freezer. Make a note and use it soon.

9. Watching portions will save money. Making extra is fine to take for lunch or a second dinner to save time; just be sure to set aside planned leftovers and not eat them all.

10. Watch weekly grocery ads. Instead of relying on the newspaper, get on the store's email list or app for specials. Get to know the people working in your favorite store, and they may be able to tell you what the planned specials are ahead of time, so you can plan menus better.

11. Split the cost and contents of warehouse-sized containers with a friend to get the good price but not struggle with storage and usage.

12. Include meatless dishes in your menu planning. Animal proteins are the most expensive part of any grocery budget. Turn to plant-based proteins such as beans to fill in and fill up.

13. Plan on more hearty, healthy yet satisfying fare such as soups, stews, and chilis that are economical, and particularly enjoyable in cooler weather.

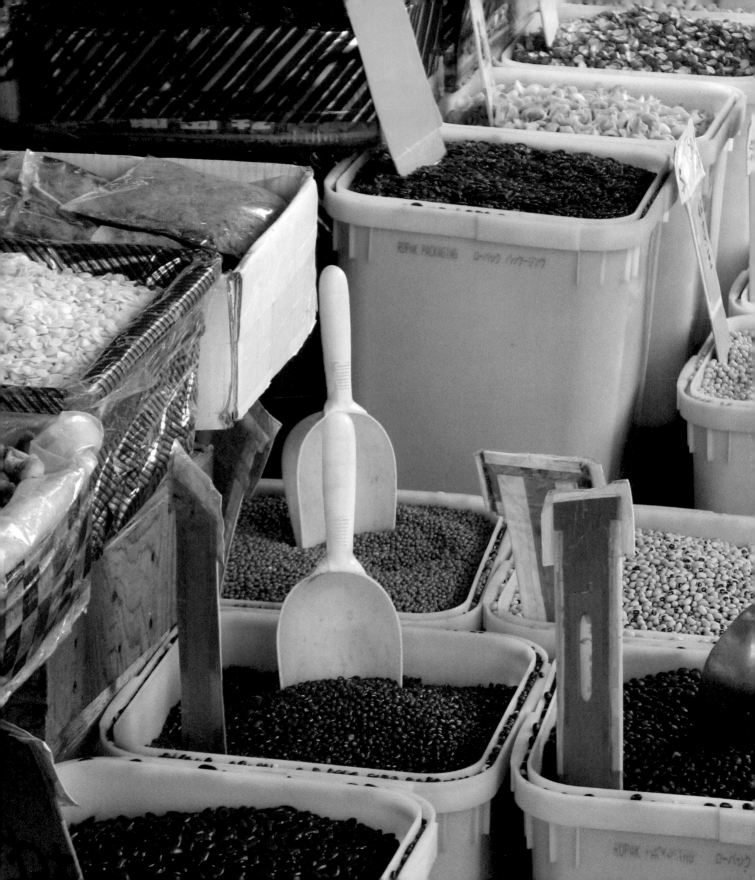

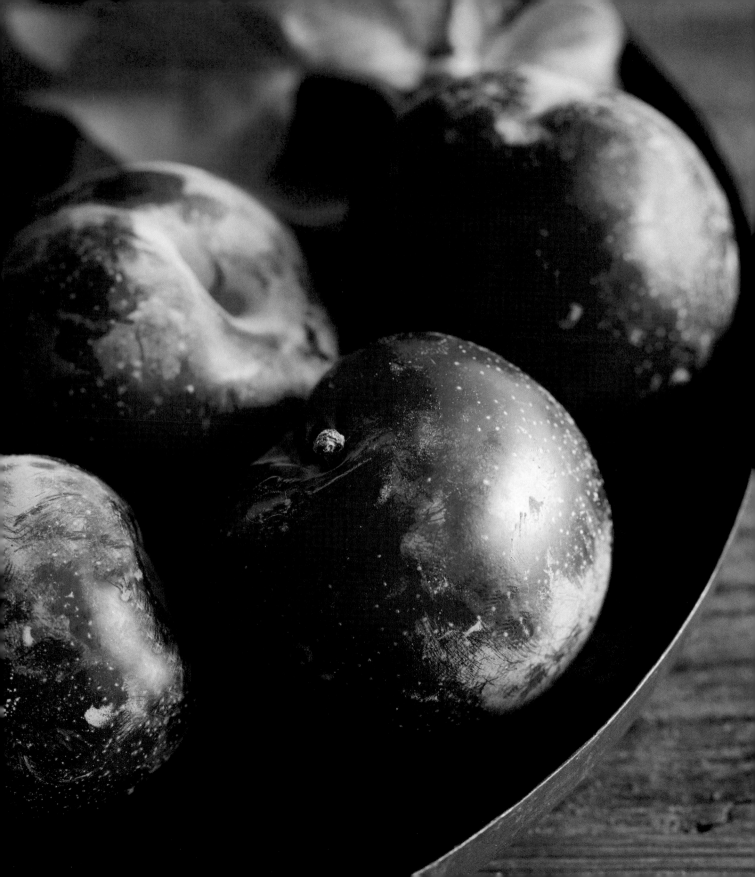

Smart Snacking

Smart snacking means choosing something with protein for balance and slow absorption and avoiding sugar. Drink plenty of water. Sometimes you are dehydrated, not hungry. Here are some great grab-and-go ideas to become a smart snacker:

- Create "snack-attack packs" to avoid food emergencies and crashing blood sugar. Include unsalted raw nuts, seeds, raw cacao nibs, goji berries, and healthy, low-sugar granola.

- Carry low-sugar fruit such as apples, pears, or berries.

- Carry a small cooler in your car for food that needs to stay cold.

- Make yogurt dip, hummus, or guacamole (see pages 173, 170, 166) with sliced raw veggies.

- Hard-boil eggs and store in the refrigerator.

- Toss together a bean salad (with olive oil, herbs, salt, pepper, or any spices such as cumin, onion, or shallot).

- Stock plain or Greek yogurt to mix with a handful of blueberries or blackberries (in a container).

- Eat cottage cheese with fresh fruit for sweetness or chopped fresh herbs and chives for a savory version. You could even add in chopped roasted red peppers. Be creative.

- Save leftover soup for lunches.

- Stock mini-packets of nut butters.

- Got a blender in your office kitchenette? Take simple ingredients for a small smoothie.

- Stock healthy jerky without added nitrates or MSG.

- Make organic air-popped popcorn.

- Buy canned wild sardines in olive oil and low-mercury tuna.

- Stash bittersweet 70 percent dark chocolate, figs, or dates for when you want a sweet treat.

Developing Healthy Portion Habits

n a country used to "super-sized" portions, it can be a surprise to understand what real, healthy portions are supposed to be. We must return to mindful eating so we can actually enjoy our meals and treat our bodies well.

Even though your parents may have demanded that you finish your plate, don't blindly feel obligated to eat everything on your plate. Stop. Think. Feel.

Allow your food to hit bottom rather than rush through a meal. You may find you eat less.

The Abundance of Whole Food

We don't count calories on The Daniel Plan. Counting calories can be a successful tool for losing weight, but The Daniel Plan focuses on overall long-term health. The emphasis is on the abundance of whole foods to impact your body and mind, helping you to cut cravings, increase your energy, and feel better. This will create long-term success.

When you consume lots of fresh vegetables and fruit, a moderate amount of lean protein, healthy whole grains, and healthy fats, your palate will begin to change, and you will be able to make better, satisfying food choices without the need to count every calorie. The things you used to eat may taste overly sweet, sugary, or artificial. You will find that the good foods your body hungers for will naturally crowd out the bad foods of the past.

When you stick to The Daniel Plan plate with half of your plate being fruit and non-starchy vegetables, one quarter lean protein, and one quarter whole grains, you can still enjoy your favorite foods—although the portions may have shifted.

Healthy eating is about abundance. It's about making smart choices and being willing to try new things. Allow bad habits to fade away as good new habits slowly

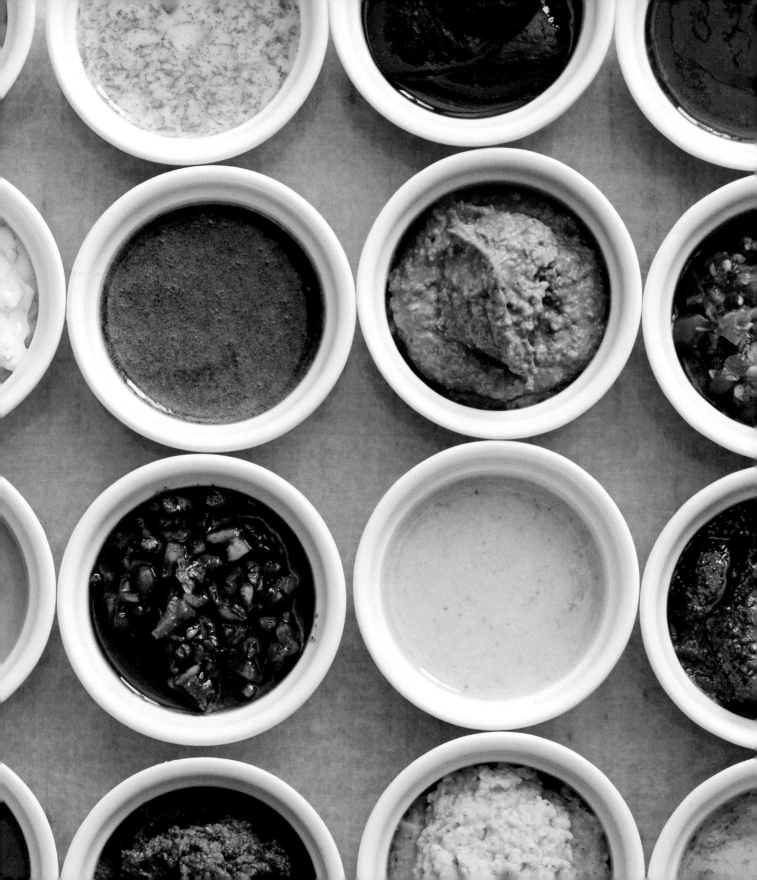

replace them. Healthy eating is about progress, not perfection. It's about the accumulation of small changes that really add up over a lifetime, versus trying to make radical changes all at once that may be hard to sustain long-term.

The Daniel Plan Plate

Understanding what portions and servings are is important to developing healthy eating habits for a lifetime. Use the following as a guideline for any meal:

- Fill half of your plate with a combination of non-starchy vegetables.

- Fill a quarter of your plate with healthy animal or vegetable protein.

- Fill a quarter of your plate with healthy starches or whole grains.

- Add a side of a low-sugar (low-glycemic) fruit.

- Drink fresh, clean water or caffeine-free herbal teas.

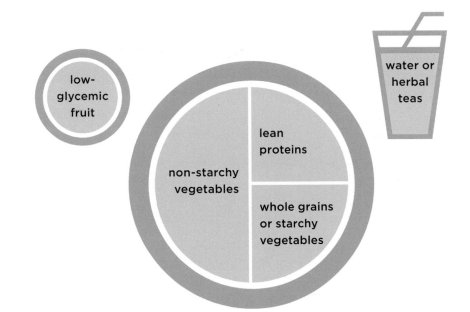

40-Day Meal Plan

To jumpstart The Daniel Plan lifestyle, we suggest you follow our 40-day meal plans in *The Daniel Plan: 40 Days to a Healthier Life*. The meal plans will help change your tastes and curb your cravings while satisfying your palate and providing you with an abundance of healthy, tasty foods.

Equivalents and Metric Conversions

The following figures are approximate metric weight and volume equivalents for common measurements provided in this cookbook. If converting to metric, use the volume amount when the U.S. measurement is given by volume (teaspoon, tablespoon, cup), and use the weight equivalent when the U.S. measurement is given by weight (ounce, pound).

U.S. Measurement	Metric Equivalent
¼ cup	60 milliliters
⅓ cup	80 milliliters
½ cup	120 milliliters
1 cup	8 fluid ounces or 236 milliliters
2 cups	460 milliliters
1 tablespoon	.5 fluid ounce or 14.8 milliliters
1 teaspoon	4.9 milliliters
1 ounce	28.35 grams
1 pound	453.59 grams
¼ inch	.6 centimeters
1 inch	2.5 centimeters

For metric equivalents, use the following general formulas:

- Ounces to grams — multiply ounces by 28.35

- Pounds to grams — multiply pounds by 453.5

- Pounds to kilograms — multiply pounds by .45

- Cups to liters — multiply cups by .24

- Fahrenheit to centigrade — subtract 32 from Fahrenheit temperature, multiply by 5, then divide by 9

The following equivalents will help you when you need to double or half a recipe.

Measurement	Equivalent
1 tablespoon	3 teaspoons
¼ cup	4 tablespoons or 12 teaspoons
½ cup	8 tablespoons
1 pint	2 cups
1 cup	8 fluid ounces
1 quart	4 cups

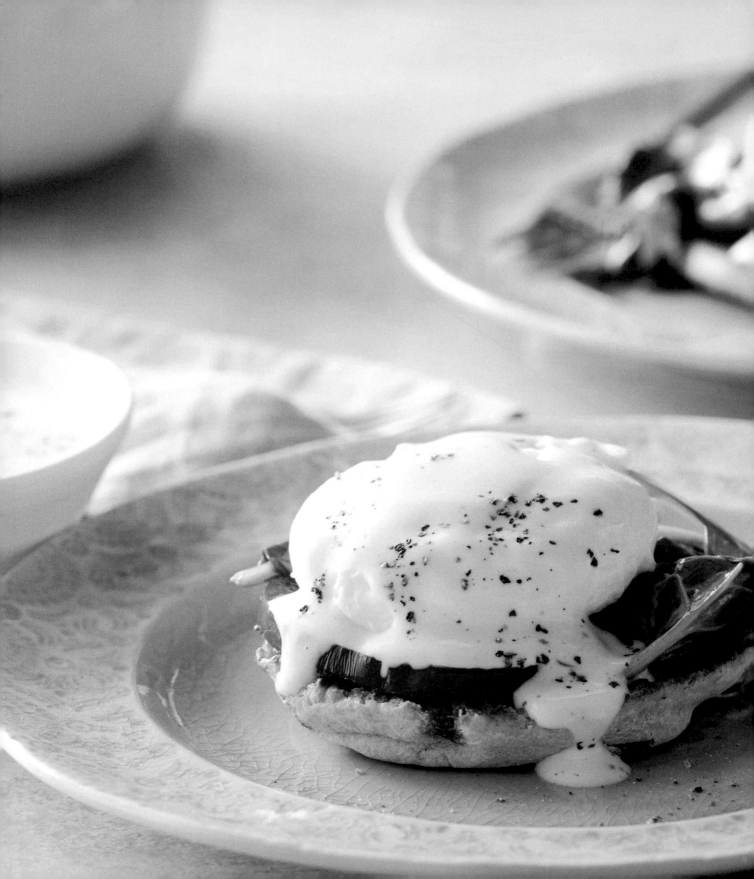

Breakfast

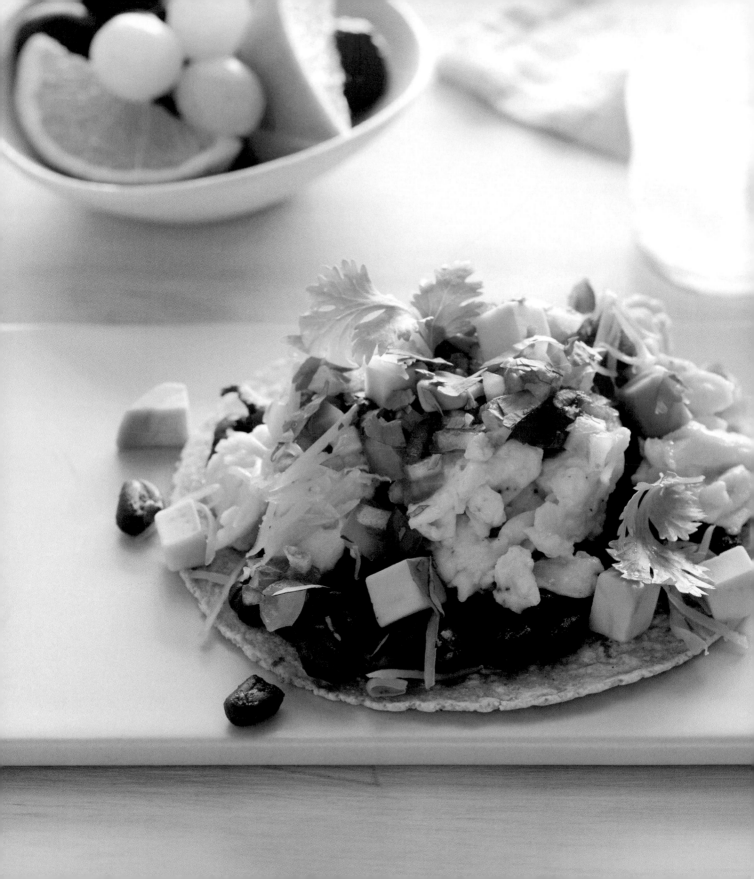

Scrambled Egg Breakfast Tostadas

1 (15-ounce) can black beans

1 teaspoon chili powder

2 teaspoons extra-virgin olive oil

¾ cup salsa

6 eggs

2 tablespoons milk (or water)

Kosher or sea salt

Black pepper

1 teaspoon olive, coconut, or avocado oil

4 organic corn tortillas

1 avocado, diced or cut into thin wedges

½ cup salsa

4 tablespoons grated cheddar cheese (omit for DF)

6–8 teaspoons fresh chopped cilantro or parsley (optional)

A colorful breakfast with Mexican flavor and flair. Black beans are high in protein and fiber; avocado adds satisfying, healthy fat; corn tortillas are gluten free; and cilantro is a detoxifying herb. A great way to start the day.

GF **4 servings**

1. Pour beans into a strainer. Rinse under cold water and drain. Place beans in a small saucepan. Add chili powder, 2 teaspoons olive oil, and ¼ cup of the salsa; stir beans and warm over medium-low heat. Cover with a lid to keep beans moist. If they get dry, add a little water or more salsa.

2. Break eggs into a medium bowl. Add milk (or water), and whisk with a little salt and pepper until frothy. Heat 1 teaspoon oil in a large nonstick sauté pan or skillet over medium-low heat.

3. Add eggs to pan. Allow eggs to cook until edges are starting to set, then push eggs into the center of the pan with a wooden spoon or spatula. Fold and stir as you scramble eggs. Cook until eggs are still a bit creamy and moist.

4. While eggs are cooking, warm tortillas for a few seconds in a pan or microwave. For a crispy base, add 1 tablespoon of oil to a sauté pan, heat until hot but not smoking, and quickly cook tortillas for a few seconds on each side until crisp. Drain on paper towels.

5. Top each tortilla with a quarter of the beans, a spoonful of eggs, ¼ avocado, salsa, 1 tablespoon cheese, and cilantro. Serve warm.

> **TIP**   Another way to heat the tortillas is directly over a low flame on a gas stove. Hold a tortilla with tongs and turn frequently until browned at the edges and warm.

Eggs Benedict

Hollandaise Sauce

½ cup organic or vegan mayonnaise

½ cup plain Greek yogurt

2 teaspoons water

1 teaspoon lemon juice

1 teaspoon Dijon mustard

2 tablespoons fresh minced dill

2 dashes hot sauce

½ teaspoon kosher or sea salt

¼ teaspoon turmeric (optional)

Eggs Benedict

4 eggs

1 quart water

2 whole wheat English muffins

1 tablespoon grape seed oil

4 ounces (4 cups or 1 bag) fresh baby spinach

1 tomato, sliced ¼-inch thick

Cracked black pepper

A classic brunch dish supposedly invented in 1894 at the Waldorf Hotel in New York City for famed Wall Street stock broker Lamuel Benedict, Eggs Benedict is traditionally made with toasted English muffins, poached eggs, Canadian bacon, and buttery hollandaise. Try this healthier version that's sure to bring a smile to anyone at your breakfast table.

2–4 servings

1. Combine all ingredients for hollandaise sauce in a small bowl. Whisk together. Set aside.

2. In a large pot, bring water to a boil. Reduce heat to a simmer. Swirl the hot water. Crack eggs individually into a small cup. Carefully drop them into the hot water. Poach eggs for about 4 minutes. Scoop out with a slotted spoon. Alternative: In a frying pan, heat grape seed oil over medium heat. Crack eggs into pan and cook 2–3 minutes on one side. Flip, and cook 1–4 minutes, depending on whether you want easy, medium, or hard yolks.

3. Toast English muffins.

4. Heat grape seed oil in sauté pan over medium heat. Sauté spinach for 1–2 minutes. Then warm the tomato slices in the pan.

5. Top each English muffin half with a warm tomato slice, ¼ of the sautéed spinach, a poached egg, and 1 tablespoon of hollandaise sauce. Sprinkle with cracked pepper.

> **TIP** Try this recipe with scrambled eggs or substitute a spicy tomato sauce for the tomato slices.

Garden Patch Omelet

2 eggs

¼ teaspoon kosher or sea salt

Dash black pepper

2 teaspoons coconut oil

¼ teaspoon minced garlic

1 cup fresh baby spinach

¼ cup diced bell pepper (red, orange, yellow)

¼ cup diced red onion

¼ cup diced tomato

1 large mushroom, thinly sliced

Dash of pepper

Filled with protein and fiber, vegetable omelets are a satisfying meal day or night. Make 1 large omelet to share or as many as you wish.

GF DF **2 servings**

1. In a bowl, whisk eggs with salt and pepper. Set aside.

2. Heat 1 teaspoon of the coconut oil over medium-high heat in a sauté or frying pan that has a lid. Add garlic, spinach, peppers, onion, tomato, and mushroom. Sauté until veggies are soft, about 5 minutes. Remove vegetables from pan. Set aside in a bowl.

3. Heat the remaining 1 teaspoon of coconut oil in the pan. Pour the eggs in the pan. Add in the veggies on top of the egg mixture, reduce heat to low, cover pan with lid. Cook for about 2 minutes. If the egg is still uncooked, cook for another minute uncovered. Fold the omelet in half.

4. Serve right away.

Optional: Chop tomatoes, avocado, and cilantro. Mix together for a breakfast side salad.

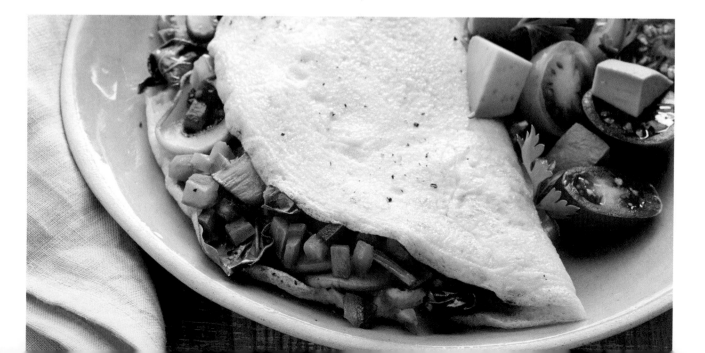

Avocado Breakfast

Simple Berry Sauce

1 cup strawberries

1 tablespoon coconut oil

1 pinch kosher or sea salt

Avocado Breakfast

4 cups mixed berries, sliced if bigger than bite-sized

2 diced avocados

1 cup simple berry sauce

Did you know that if you eat well for breakfast, you are more likely to eat well all day long? This is a simple, easy breakfast dish that can also provide some variety in your breakfast routine. This dish is all plant-based.

GF DF V **2 servings**

1. Combine all sauce ingredients in a blender and blend well. Transfer to a storage container for use for up to five days. Store in the refrigerator.

2. In a small mixing bowl, toss together half the berries and half the avocado lightly with half the berry sauce until well coated. Repeat with remaining berries, avocado, and sauce.

Optional: Serve over a half of avocado.

> **TIP** As a variation throughout your week, top the avocado breakfast with the simple berry sauce and fresh superfoods or shredded coconut for more flavor and further nutritional value.

Food as Medicine

This dish offers a balanced approach to a plant-based breakfast, providing essential fatty acids for brain health and morning endurance, as well as antioxidants and fiber. For additional protein, consider adding granola, seeds, or chopped nuts.

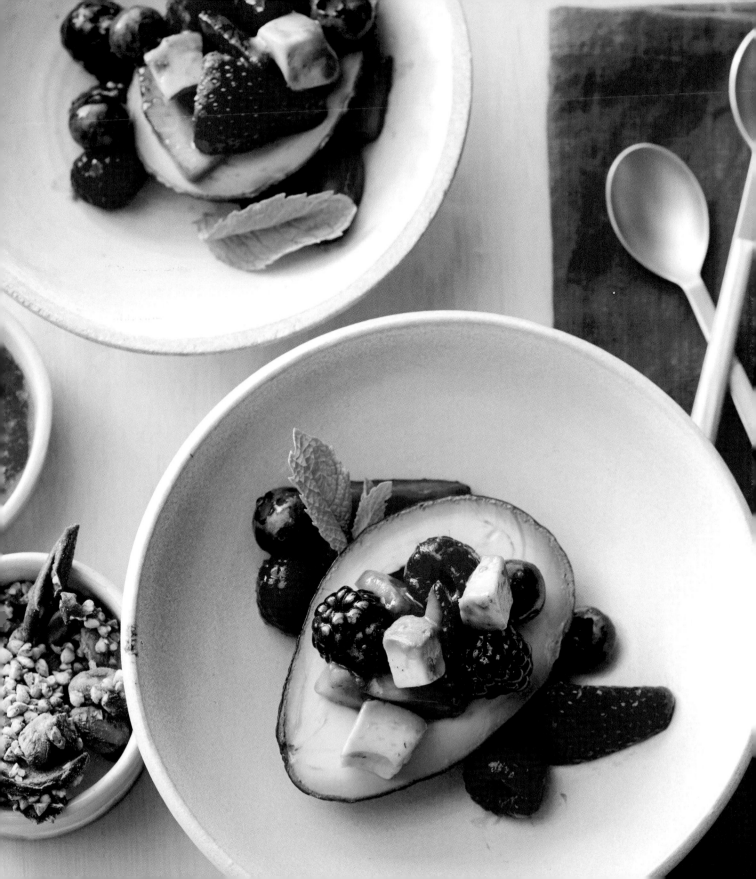

Buckwheat Buttermilk Pancakes

1¾ cups (8½ ounces) whole grain buckwheat flour

1½ teaspoons baking powder

¾ teaspoon baking soda

½ teaspoon kosher or sea salt

2 large eggs

3 tablespoons coconut oil, plus extra for topping

2 tablespoons raw honey

1 teaspoon pure vanilla extract

2½ cups buttermilk

Coconut or grape seed oil

Blackberries for garnish (optional)

Buckwheat is not wheat, but a fruit seed related to the rhubarb plant. Buckwheat is gluten free and high in protein and fiber with an earthy, nutty flavor and a rich brown color. Enjoy these hearty, high-energy pancakes topped with superfood Blackberry Sauce (page 71) instead of syrup.

GF Eighteen 4-inch pancakes

1. Preheat oven to 200°, and place a rimmed baking sheet inside the oven to keep cooked pancakes warm.

2. In a medium bowl, whisk together flour, baking soda, baking powder, and salt.

3. In a small bowl, whisk eggs, coconut oil, honey, and vanilla until smooth. Whisk in buttermilk. Don't worry about small lumps from the coconut oil. Pour the liquid ingredients into the dry mixture, and whisk together. Batter will be thick.

4. Heat a large nonstick griddle over medium heat. Reduce heat to medium-low and grease with oil. Using a ¼ cup measure, pour batter in circles onto hot griddle. Allow batter to cook until small bubbles start to form and break on the top. Then carefully flip the pancake. The top of the pancake should be golden brown.

5. Cook pancakes about 1 minute on the other side, and then move them to the baking sheet and set in the oven. Cover with a clean kitchen towel while you make the rest of the pancakes.

6. Serve pancakes with a drizzle of melted coconut oil, blackberries, and Blackberry Sauce.

Blackberry Sauce

2 (10-ounce) bags frozen (or fresh) blackberries

2 teaspoons raw honey

This sauce is perfect over buckwheat pancakes but works equally well as a dessert sauce. It is great swirled into plain Greek yogurt for a snack or quick breakfast. It is easy to make year-round with frozen berries of any kind. Use fresh berries when they are in season. Extra sauce freezes well.

2 cups

1. Thaw berries in the refrigerator overnight or in a small saucepan over low heat. Break them apart as they thaw.

2. Puree berries in a blender until smooth. Pour the berry puree into a sieve or strainer set over a bowl. With the back of a ladle, press the berries through the sieve until all that is left in the sieve is seeds. Discard seeds.

3. Stir honey into berry puree.

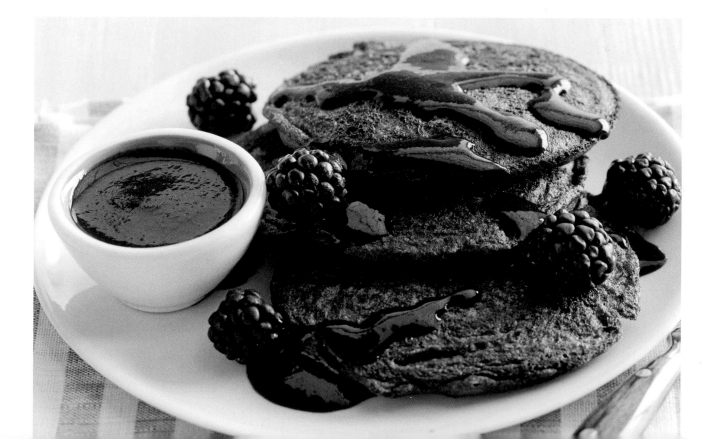

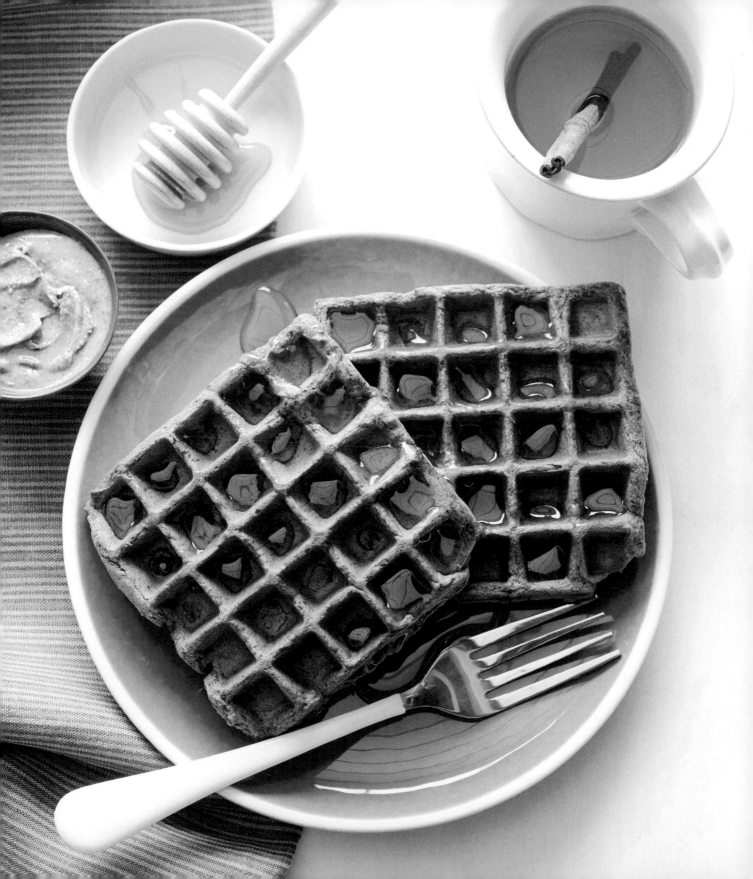

Gluten-Free Pumpkin Waffles

1 cup rice flour

1½ cups all-purpose
gluten-free flour mix

⅛ cup flax seeds

2 tablespoons cinnamon

1 teaspoon baking powder

1 teaspoon baking soda

1 teaspoon kosher
or sea salt

8 ounces pumpkin puree
(canned or fresh)

1 cup almond milk

2 tablespoons extra-virgin
olive oil or coconut oil,
plus extra for greasing

Raw honey (optional)

Waffles are a kid pleaser for sure, and these waffles can double as bread or a Daniel Plan–approved dessert! For breakfast, we recommend topping the waffles with almond butter, bananas, and a sprinkle of cinnamon for a nutritional power punch.

GF **DF**   4 servings

1. Preheat a waffle iron to medium.

2. In a medium mixing bowl, whisk together the flours, baking powder, baking soda, and salt until combined.

3. In another medium bowl, combine pumpkin puree, milk, and oil. Mix well.

4. Pour the liquid mixture into the dry mixture, and whisk together until you have a silky texture.

5. Lightly coat the waffle iron with olive or coconut oil. According to manufacturer's instructions, pour batter onto the bottom portion of the waffle iron. Close the waffle iron. When the steam minimizes from the sides of your waffle iron, check the waffle to see if it is ready. It should be crispy and light.

6. Keep waffles in a warm oven until ready to serve. Drizzle with honey before serving.

Food as Medicine

Pumpkin is a great source of vitamin A, vitamin C, and fiber. Pumpkin, which is rich in carotenoids, can help lower your risk of high blood pressure and cardiovascular disease.

Hearty Apple Oatmeal

2 cups water

1 cup old-fashioned rolled oats (gluten-free)

¼ teaspoon kosher or sea salt

4 tablespoons chopped apples

Pinch of stevia extract or 1 teaspoon pure maple syrup

2 scoops of unsweetened protein powder (optional)

4 teaspoons chopped walnuts or pecans

¼ teaspoon cinnamon or pumpkin pie spice

Oatmeal is a classic go-to breakfast option that will energize you and keep you full for hours. Lower the glycemic index by adding nuts and seeds. Get creative with it by adding your favorite spices or alternative milk. Steel-cut oats are nice as well. Just follow package directions for appropriate cooking times.

GF **2 servings**

1. In a small saucepan, bring the water to a boil. Stir in the oats and salt. As soon as the water begins to boil again, reduce the heat to a simmer.

2. Cook for about 5 minutes, stirring occasionally or until oats reach desired consistency.

3. Add chopped apple, stevia or maple syrup, protein powder, nuts, and spice to the oatmeal. Mix well.

Alternative: Easy Overnight Steel-Cut Oats   If you prefer steel-cut oats, cook them a bit the night before. In a 2-quart saucepan with a tight-fitting lid, heat 2 teaspoons of coconut oil. Add 1 cup of steel-cut oats, and cook the oats for a few minutes, until they smell toasty. Add 3 cups water, and bring to a full boil. Turn off the heat, cover the pan, and remove from the heat. Allow the oats to stand overnight on the stove. They turn creamy and wonderful while you are sleeping.

Oats and Gluten?

Oats are naturally gluten free; however, many oats are grown or processed near other gluten-containing grains, such as wheat, barley, or rye. To avoid gluten, be sure to look for gluten-free oats that have not been cross-contaminated.

Blueberry French Toast

1 pound fresh blueberries

1 tablespoon raw honey or pure maple syrup

1 tablespoon fresh lemon juice

¼ teaspoon pure vanilla extract

Coconut oil

6 eggs

½ cup coconut milk

8 slices thick whole wheat or multigrain bread

2 bananas, sliced

4 whole strawberries, sliced

½ cup unsweetened coconut, toasted

2 tablespoons chopped almonds

Surprised we're encouraging you to eat French toast? Many breakfast classics can be made healthy with just a few changes. This recipe is dairy free and can also be gluten free by using a gluten-free bread.

DF **4 servings**

1. Put blueberries, honey, and lemon juice in a small saucepan over medium heat. Bring to a boil. Lower heat and simmer for 10 minutes until syrupy. Turn off heat, add vanilla extract, and set aside.

2. Heat coconut oil in nonstick frying pan or griddle over medium heat.

3. Beat eggs and coconut milk in a large, shallow bowl. Dip each slice of bread in the egg batter to coat both sides.

4. Cook each slice of bread until golden brown, about 2 minutes on each side.

5. Place two slices of toast on each plate, pour a quarter of the blueberry sauce over French toast. Arrange banana slices and strawberries on top. Sprinkle with toasted coconut and raw almonds.

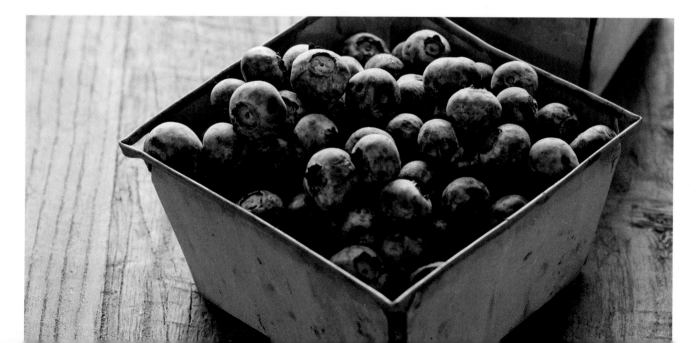

Whole Foods Protein Shake

1 cup frozen blueberries

2 tablespoons almond butter

2 tablespoons pumpkin seeds

2 tablespoons chia seeds

2 tablespoons hemp seeds

4 raw walnuts

4 raw Brazil nuts

½ avocado

1 tablespoon extra-virgin coconut oil

1 cup unsweetened almond or hemp milk

1 cup water

Since smoothies are easy to digest, your body can use the nutrients in them quickly and easily. Use a smoothie in place of a meal or as a side for a quick shot of additional nutrients. This recipe is one of Dr. Hyman's go-to morning choices. The original version of this shake appeared in *The Blood Sugar Solution Cookbook* by Mark Hyman, M.D.

(GF) (DF) (V) **2 servings**

Combine all the ingredients in a blender. Cover with lid. Blend on high speed until smooth. Be sure to add enough water so that the smoothie is drinkable but still thick (total liquid should be about an inch or two above the other ingredients).

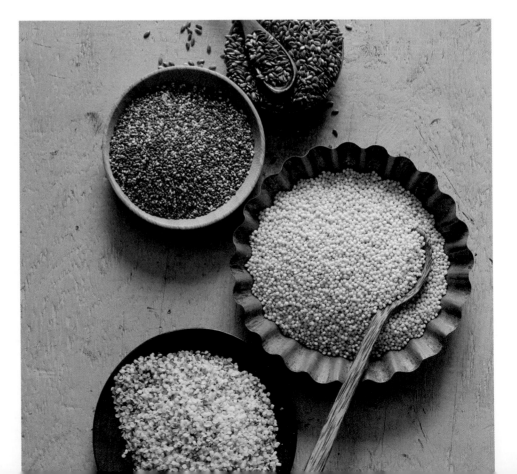

Very Cherry Smoothie

1 cup organic pitted frozen cherries

8 ounces almond milk, unsweetened

1 cup fresh baby spinach

2–3 kale leaves

¼ cup raw nuts

1 tablespoon chia seeds

1 scoop vanilla protein powder

1 tablespoon freeze-dried greens (available in health food stores)

1 dropper full vanilla stevia extract

Dr. Amen Favorite

Stock up on frozen fruit so you can enjoy your favorite summer flavors year-round. Dr. Amen likes to jumpstart his day with this drink. The original version of this smoothie appeared in *The Omni Diet* by Tana Amen, B.S.N., R.N.

GF **2 servings**

1. Put all ingredients into blender. Cover with lid. Blend on high until smooth and creamy.

2. Add water or almond milk as needed to achieve desired consistency. Serve immediately.

Food as Medicine

Experiment with hemp, chia, and flax seeds; they are rich in omega-3 fats, minerals, and fiber.

Berry Protein Smoothie

3 cups unsweetened almond milk (hemp, coconut, soy, or oat)

2 small bananas (or 1 large)

1 cup unsweetened frozen berries of choice

2 scoops of vanilla protein powder

A little stevia or 1 teaspoon of honey (optional, try it first without)

Smoothies whip up in less than 5 minutes, are customizable for individual taste and nutritional preference, and are transportable for busy mornings. The amount of protein powder you need may vary by the brand you buy. Check the label for the recommended serving size.

GF **2 servings**

Place all ingredients in a blender. Cover with lid. Blend on high until the smoothie is smooth and creamy. Serve immediately.

TIP Ice is optional in a smoothie. If you prefer yours frosty, add ½ cup of ice, then all the fruits. Finish by adding in the greens and any superfoods.

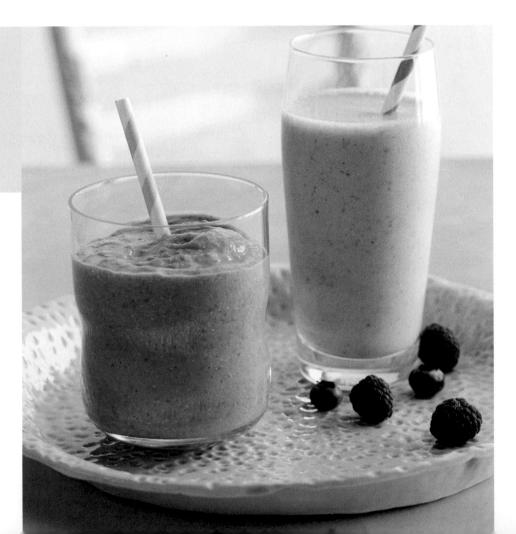

Green Smoothie

1 cup almond milk,
coconut water, or apple
cider

2 cups fresh fruit
(peaches, pineapple,
mango, or berries)

2 small bananas or
1 avocado

2 cups fresh raw spinach,
kale, or red chard

1–2 drops stevia (optional)

4 tablespoons chia seeds
or hemp seeds (optional,
adds 12–14g protein)

Why a green smoothie? That's a perfectly good question with a variety of answers, but here are just a few to get you started! First, it's a great way to get in your greens without having a salad. Second, adding greens to your smoothie adds nutritional benefits such as fiber and minerals. Plus, a smoothie is a grab-and-go meal in a cup.

GF DF **2 servings**

Place all ingredients in a blender. Cover with lid. Blend the mixture on high until all greens are well combined. You should have a creamy smooth mixture, almost as thick as a milkshake! Serve immediately.

TIP There are many options for protein powder. Find them at health food, grocery, and vitamin stores as well as online. You will find whey (from cow's milk) and egg white powders for animal-based protein. Plant-based protein options are blended from pea, brown rice, cranberry, hemp or other seeds, beans, sea algae, and more. A plant-based protein powder will allow you to transform any of these smoothies to dairy free and vegan. Look for a version that is not sweetened with sugar and is without preservatives. Buy a sample size or small container to start. Once you find one you like, buy in a larger quantity to save money.

Alternative Milks

Alternative milks are a great substitute or upgrade from standard dairy milk. The tendency when swapping out milk is to purchase boxed milks; however, it's simple to make a number of alternative milks at home each week that can save you money.

All of these milks can be spiced up however you prefer. We recommend keeping them basic so they are easily adaptable for use in multiple dishes throughout your week. Once you learn the technique, apply it for all sorts of nuts and seeds. **GF** **DF** **V** **4 servings**

Raw Nut Milk

1 cup raw almonds
or nuts

Alternative:
4 tablespoons raw
almond butter

4–6 cups water

TIP Fold the almond pulp into recipes for baked goods or dry it in a dehydrator and grind down to a flour once dry.

1. Cover the raw nuts with water in a glass bowl. Let sit for 4–6 hours. This releases the enzyme inhibitors and creates enzyme-active plump almonds to milk in your blender. This step is optional, but creates a nice thick milk that will be easy to digest.

2. Drain the nuts to remove the soak water and enzyme inhibitors. Place the nuts in the blender with 4 cups of fresh water. Blend on high for 1 to 2 minutes. The mixture will be naturally full of pulp at this point and thick.

3. Line a glass jar that can catch at least 24 ounces of liquid with a cheesecloth or nut milk bag. Grip the cloth well with your hands.

4. Slowly pour the nut mixture a little at a time into the cloth or bag. Stop when your hands begin to fill up around the bag or cloth. Then squeeze out the thick creamy milk into the glass container, leaving behind the pulp. Repeat this step until the entire mixture has been "milked."

5. Place the pulp in a storage container (see tip).

6. Store for up to 5 days in the refrigerator. Stir or shake prior to use.

Shortcut: Use pre-ground almond or other nut butter. Simply combine the butter and water into a blender, and blend on high very well. Store for up to three days in the refrigerator, and shake before using.

Coconut Milk

1 cup unsweetened shredded coconut

Alternative: fresh coconut flesh

4–6 cups water

Pinch of kosher or sea salt

1. Soak the shredded coconut in water for about an hour. If using fresh coconut, no soaking is necessary.

2. Strain the coconut, and discard the soaking water. Place 4 cups of fresh water and coconut into a blender. Blend on high until well combined.

3. Add a pinch of salt to bring out the coconut flavor. Store for up to 3 days in the refrigerator. Shake or stir prior to use.

TIP   Find nut milk bags online and in health food stores.

Hemp or Chia Seed Milk

½ cup hemp or chia seeds

4 cups water

1. If using chia seeds, soak them for about 20 minutes prior to using. Discard soaking water.

2. Add the seeds and water to a blender. Cover with lid. Blend on high until well combined. It should be rich and creamy.

3. Store this milk in the refrigerator for up to 5 days. Shake milk prior to each use.

Alternative: Both types of seed milk are delicious with cinnamon or a drop of stevia. One trick is to add a pinch of salt so you can bring out the natural sweetness of the milk.

Food as Medicine
Coconut makes a solid alternative to nuts, seeds, and dairy. The essential fatty acids in coconut fill important nutritional components of The Daniel Plan.

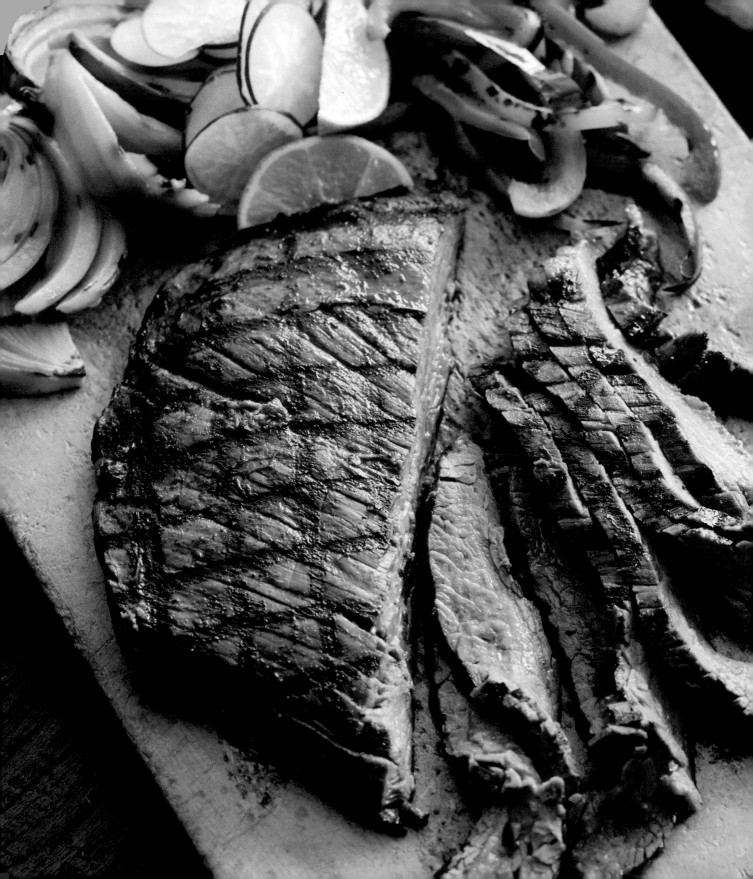

American Classics

BBQ Chicken Pizza

Venetian Style Arugula Pizza

Goat Cheese and Turkey Bacon Pizza

Honey Wheat Pizza Crust

Gluten-Free Pizza Crust

Herbed Turkey Burgers

Quinoa-Lentil Veggie Burgers

Lemon-Dijon Sauce

Caramelized Onion Burgers

Turkey Sloppy Joes

Grilled Spicy Fish Tacos ✓

Mango-Jalapeno Salsa

Roast Chicken Tacos ✓

Creamy Chipotle-Lime Sauce

Veggie Tacos ✓

◄ Kicking and Screaming Steak Fajitas

Pasta Primaverde

Spaghetti and Meatballs

Savory Spaghetti Sauce

Mac and Cheese

Five-Veggie Lasagna

Zucchini Pasta

BBQ Chicken Pizza

1 honey wheat or gluten-free pizza crust (pages 88–89)

3 ounces organic BBQ sauce

1 cup thinly sliced grilled or roasted chicken

½ cup thinly sliced red onion

½ cup diced pineapple (optional)

½ cup fresh cilantro leaves

3 ounces shredded mozzarella cheese

One of the most popular pizzas in America is BBQ Chicken Pizza. Here is a healthy version sure to please any BBQ lover.

One 12-inch pizza

1. Pre-heat oven to 450°.

2. Spread BBQ sauce over crust. Arrange chicken slices on crust. Top with mozzarella cheese. Sprinkle with red onion strips and pineapple.

3. Bake on pizza stone or cookie sheet for 10–12 minutes.

4. Remove from oven, and spread cilantro over top of the hot pizza.

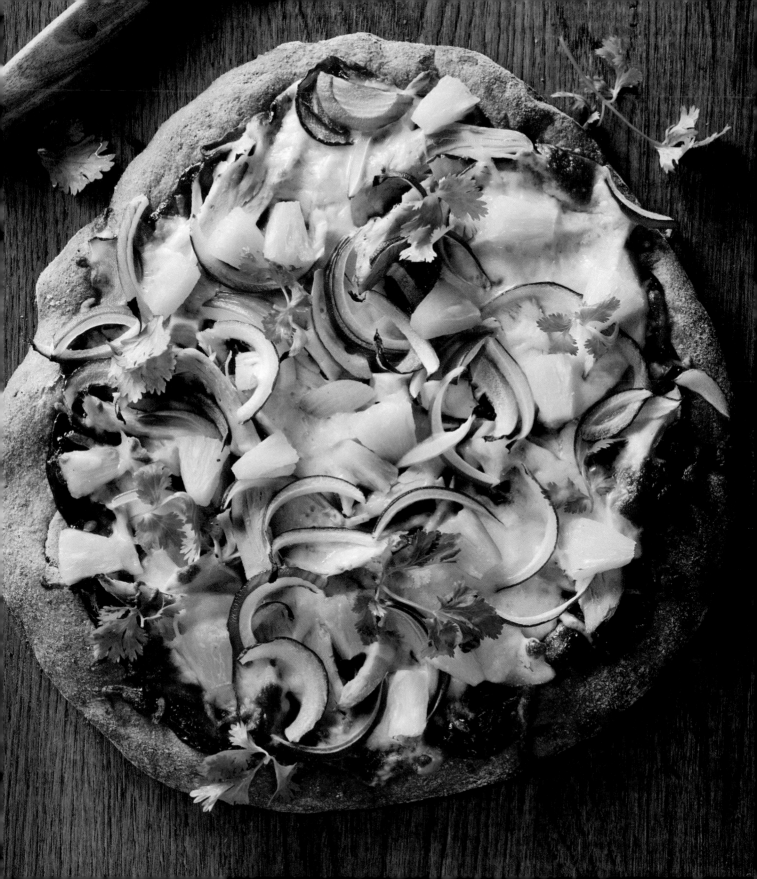

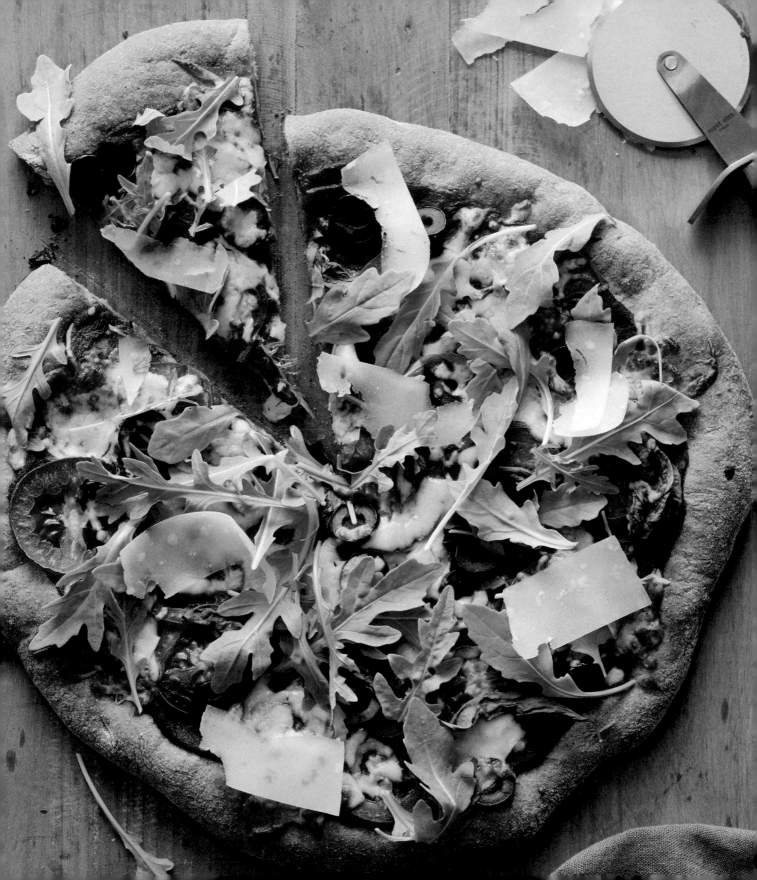

Venetian Style Arugula Pizza

1 honey whole wheat pizza crust (page 88)

½ cup (3 ounces) organic pizza sauce

1 Roma tomato, thinly sliced

¼ cup sliced black olives

12 fresh basil leaves

½ cup (3 ounces) shredded mozzarella cheese

1 cup baby arugula

¼ cup shaved Parmesan cheese

This is a unique take on pizza. The arugula adds a peppery bite that we know you'll love! **One 12-inch pizza**

1. Preheat oven to 450°.

2. Spread pizza sauce over honey wheat crust. Lay tomato slices on crust, and cover with black olives and basil leaves. Top with mozzarella cheese.

3. Bake on pizza stone for 10–12 minutes. Remove from oven, and spread arugula over top of the hot pizza. Sprinkle with Parmesan cheese.

Goat Cheese and Turkey Bacon Pizza

1 (12-inch) gluten-free crust (page 89)

⅓ cup organic pizza sauce

1 small onion, thinly sliced, separated into rings

4–6 strips turkey bacon, cut into ¼-inch strips

1 pear (or apple), peeled, thinly sliced

2 ounces crumbled goat cheese

2 ounces shredded mozzarella cheese

1 tablespoon pine nuts, toasted (optional)

¼ cup chopped fresh basil

½ teaspoon crushed red pepper

A healthy gourmet twist on traditional meat pizzas, the flavors will seem familiar but new. **GF** **One 12-inch pizza**

1. Preheat oven to 450°.

2. Spread pizza sauce over gluten-free crust. Arrange onion, turkey bacon, and pears on sauce. Top with cheeses.

3. Bake on pizza stone for 12–14 minutes. Remove from oven and top with pine nuts, basil, and red pepper flakes.

Honey Wheat Pizza Crust

2 cups whole wheat flour

1 package active dry yeast
or instant yeast

¾ teaspoon kosher
or sea salt

1 cup warm water
(105–115°)

1 tablespoon olive or
grape seed oil

1 tablespoon raw honey

¼ cup grated Parmesan
cheese

One 12-inch crust

1. In large mixing bowl, combine whole wheat flour, yeast, and salt. Blend in water, oil, raw honey, and cheese. Stir by hand vigorously until all ingredients are well mixed, about 3 minutes. Or in a stand mixer with a dough hook, mix dough until smooth about 1 minute.

2. Cover with plastic wrap, and let rise to double in size, about 1½–2 hours.

3. Preheat oven to 450°.

4. Sprinkle a dusting of flour over a 12 × 12-inch clean, smooth surface. Place the dough on the floured smooth surface. Use your hand or rolling pin to press the dough down forming a flat 12-inch circle about ½-inch thick.

5. Add pizza sauce of your choice and your favorite pizza toppings.

6. Bake on a pizza stone in oven 10–12 minutes, or until crust is golden brown and toppings are done.

Gluten-Free Pizza Crust

1 packet active dry yeast

1 cup warm water
(105–115˚)

2 tablespoons extra-virgin olive oil, plus extra for greasing the bowl

1 teaspoon raw honey

1 egg white

2½ cups gluten-free flour mix (plus extra for rolling out the pizza)

1 teaspoon kosher or sea salt

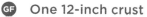 **One 12-inch crust**

1. Combine yeast and warm water in the bowl of a stand mixer fitted with a dough hook. Let sit until yeast begins to foam and float on surface of the water, about 10 minutes.

2. Add oil, honey, and egg. Mix well.

3. Preheat oven to 450°.

4. In a separate bowl, mix together flour and salt. With the mixer running, slowly add flour mixture, a few tablespoons at a time. Mix until a smooth dough forms, about 10 minutes.

5. Transfer dough to a bowl coated with some olive oil; cover with plastic wrap. Let sit at room temperature for 1 hour or until the dough doubles in size.

6. Divide dough into 2 balls. Working with 1 ball at a time, dust dough with flour. Roll dough into a 12-inch round about ¼-inch thick. Repeat with remaining dough ball or freeze remaining dough ball for up to 3 months (wrap it tightly in plastic wrap and then aluminum foil to keep the plastic wrap secure).

7. Add pizza sauce of your choice and your favorite pizza toppings.

8. Bake on a pizza stone in oven 10–12 minutes, or until crust is golden brown and toppings are done.

TIP Make your own gluten-free flour mix by combining 1 cup rice flour, ¾ cup tapioca flour, and ¾ cup garbanzo bean flour.

Herbed Turkey Burgers

1¼ pounds lean ground turkey

2 tablespoons finely chopped fresh parsley

2 tablespoons finely chopped fresh chives

4 teaspoons extra-virgin olive oil

1½ tablespoons coarse or whole grain Dijon mustard

3 tablespoons bread crumbs (whole wheat panko or gluten-free)

2–3 large cloves garlic, minced

4 whole wheat or gluten-free buns

4 large tomato slices

4 large leaves dark green lettuce

Horseradish sauce and Dijon to dress buns (optional)

When shopping for ground turkey, read labels for the fat to lean ratio. Choose an 85%–90% lean grind, dark meat if possible, for best flavor. Some dark ground turkey is higher in fat because turkey skin is ground into the meat. You may want to ask the butcher to grind some for you. To grind your own, use a manual meat grinder or a standing mixer with a grinding attachment. (DF) **4 servings**

1. Place turkey, herbs, oil, mustard, bread crumbs, and garlic into a medium bowl. Mix gently with your hands until thoroughly combined.

2. Divide turkey mixture into 4 equal portions. Roll into balls, and then flatten into burger patties. Patties can be refrigerated at this point for a few hours or grilled right away.

3. Cook burgers in a nonstick grill or frying pan or on an outdoor grill. Place patties on the grill, and cook until one side has golden grill marks and feels firm, about 7–9 minutes. Flip burgers and cover with a lid or a small aluminum pan, and cook until burgers are firm and reach an internal temperature of 160°–165°. Do not overcook or press on burgers while they are cooking; you want juicy burgers.

4. Spread the buns with a little horseradish sauce and/or Dijon mustard, top with lettuce and tomatoes. Add burgers.

> **TIP** Homemade bread crumbs taste the best and are easy to make. Cut crusts from a few slices of bread (leftover bread is perfect, and gluten-free bread works just as well). Tear remaining bread into pieces, then pulse in a food processor until fine. Spread bread crumbs on a rimmed baking sheet. Bake at 350° for a few minutes until dry and toasted. Cool before using. Crumbs will keep several months refrigerated or frozen.

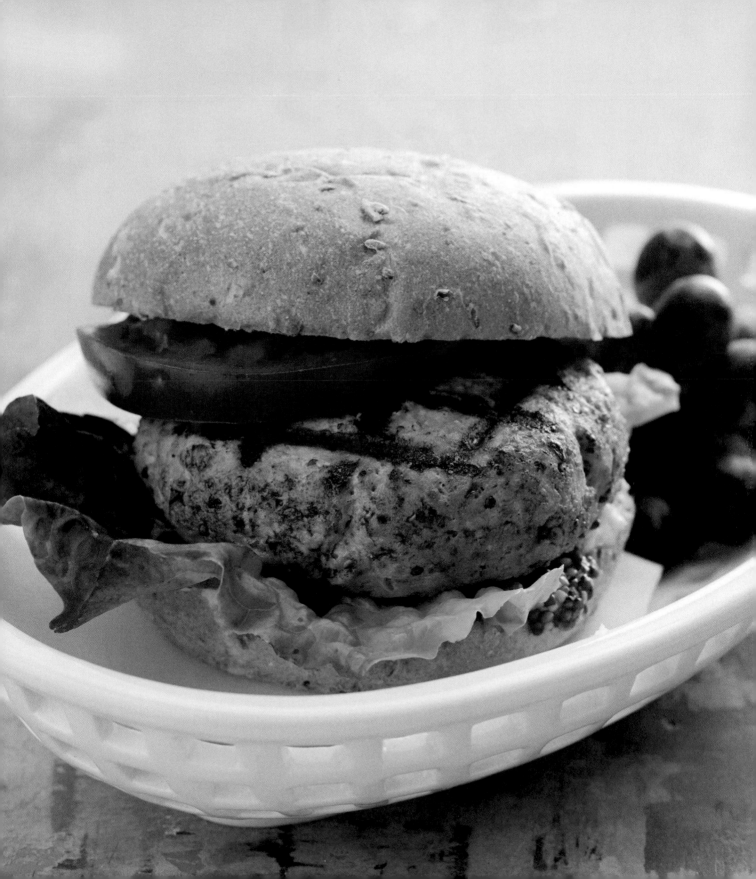

Quinoa-Lentil Veggie Burgers

6 ounces brown or white mushrooms

2 tablespoons extra-virgin olive oil

½ cup chopped onion

3 large garlic cloves, minced

1 tablespoon wheat-free tamari or soy sauce

¼ cup chopped fresh parsley

2 tablespoons chopped fresh oregano

¼ teaspoon black pepper

1 (15-ounce) can cooked lentils, rinsed and drained

1 large egg, beaten

1 cup cooked quinoa

½ cup (or more) bread crumbs (gluten-free or whole wheat)

4 tablespoons grated Parmesan cheese (omit for DF)

4 teaspoons coarse or whole grain Dijon mustard

5 slices mozzarella or Jack cheese (omit for DF)

5 whole grain or gluten-free buns

Lettuce leaves

5 large slices tomato

These generously sized veggie burgers are a nice change from meat burgers. Use gluten-free bread crumbs and buns for a gluten-free meal. Add lettuce and tomatoes for more fresh flavor. Tri-color or red quinoa adds nice color, but white quinoa will work fine. These patties will not work well directly on a grill because they are too soft. **5 servings**

1. Pulse mushrooms in the food processor until finely chopped, or chop by hand.

2. Heat 1 tablespoon of the olive oil in a sauté or frying pan over medium heat. Cook onion until soft. Add garlic and tamari. Cook 1 more minute.

3. Add mushrooms. Cook until mushrooms release their moisture and are almost dry. Add parsley, oregano, and black pepper. Add lentils, and stir well.

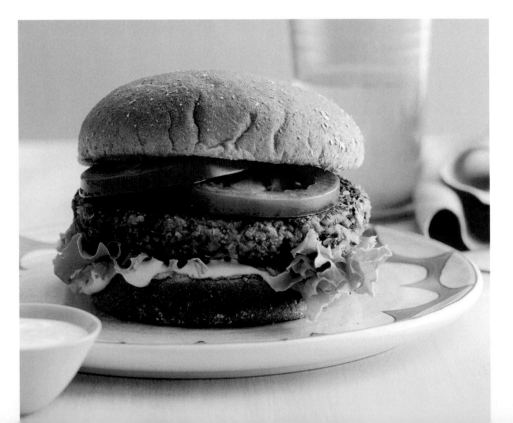

4. Put lentil mixture into food processor, and pulse mixture to grind, about 7 times.

5. In a large bowl, combine mushroom-lentil mixture with beaten egg, quinoa, bread crumbs, Parmesan, and mustard. Mix well. Moisture level of mixture may vary with the type of bread crumbs used. It should be very moist, but not be wet. If it feels wet, add bread crumbs 1 tablespoon at a time.

6. Divide into 5 portions, about a generous ½ cup each. Roll each portion into a ball, then flatten to form patties about 3½ inches across and ¾-inch thick. Place patties on a flat plate or rimmed baking sheet, cover with plastic film and refrigerate for 30 minutes or overnight.

7. Heat the remaining tablespoon of olive oil in a large nonstick pan or flat griddle over medium heat. Add patties, and cook until browned on one side, about 5–6 minutes. Carefully turn patties and cook another 5–6 minutes on the other side. Optional: Top with cheese so it melts the last minute of cooking.

8. Toast buns and dress with Lemon-Dijon sauce (below), lettuce, and tomato.

Lemon-Dijon Sauce

4 tablespoons organic or vegan mayonnaise

1 tablespoon coarse or whole grain Dijon mustard

1 garlic clove, minced

Juice of one lemon

Kosher or sea salt and black pepper

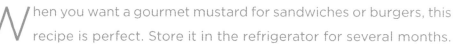

When you want a gourmet mustard for sandwiches or burgers, this recipe is perfect. Store it in the refrigerator for several months.

GF **6 tablespoons**

Whisk ingredients in a small bowl and refrigerate.

Caramelized Onion Burgers

2 teaspoons extra-virgin olive oil

4 cups sliced sweet onions (2–3 onions)

4 cloves garlic, minced

1 tablespoon balsamic vinegar

1 teaspoon kosher or sea salt

¼ teaspoon cayenne pepper

1 pound 90% lean ground beef or buffalo

2 tablespoons tomato paste

2 tablespoons fresh chopped parsley

½ teaspoon black pepper

4 gluten-free buns (optional)

Lettuce leaves

Onions are one of the world's healthiest foods. Onions are anti-bacterial and anti-microbial, help prevent colon cancer, lower blood sugar, and help with diabetes and sinus relief. You can even squeeze onion juice on a bee sting for immediate pain relief. Go figure.

GF **DF** **4 servings**

1. Heat olive oil in a nonstick skillet over medium-low heat. Add onions and garlic; cook, stirring occasionally, until the onions are very tender and golden, about 15 minutes.

2. Stir in vinegar, ½ teaspoon of the salt, and cayenne pepper. Set aside and keep warm.

3. Preheat the grill or broiler to high. Combine the beef, tomato paste, parsley, the remaining salt, and pepper in a medium bowl, knead thoroughly with your hands.

4. Shape into 4 patties about ¾-inch thick. Grill or broil on a lightly oiled rack until browned and cooked through, about 5 minutes per side.

5. Serve patties on buns or wrap with lettuce, top with the caramelized onions and lettuce.

OPTIONAL   Try this recipe with ground turkey or chicken. Top with Homemade Ketchup (see page 226).

Turkey Sloppy Joes

2 tablespoons vegetable oil

1 pound ground turkey, beef, or lamb

½ cup diced onion

½ cup diced green pepper

3 cloves garlic, minced

1 tablespoon Dijon or yellow mustard

1 tablespoon chili powder

¼ cup organic or Homemade Ketchup (page 226)

1 (15-ounce) can no-salt-added tomato sauce

1 tablespoon organic BBQ sauce

2–3 drops of liquid stevia extract (optional)

Parmesan cheese (omit for DF)

Whole grain or gluten-free buns or zucchini boats

Sloppy Joes originally consisted of ground beef, onions, tomato sauce or ketchup, and other seasonings, served on a hamburger bun. Try this Daniel Plan version of an American classic.   **4–6 servings**

1. Heat oil in a large frying pan over medium heat.

2. Brown raw turkey, onion, and green pepper.

3. Add all the other ingredients and mix well. Bring to a boil. Reduce heat to a simmer. Cover and simmer 30 minutes.

4. Serve on toasted buns or in zucchini halves (see optional).

OPTIONAL
Here's a twist! Try stuffing a zucchini with the Sloppy Joe mix. Cut a zucchini in half lengthwise, scoop out the seeds to make a "canoe." Top it off with a bit of Parmesan cheese, and bake it at 400° till golden brown.

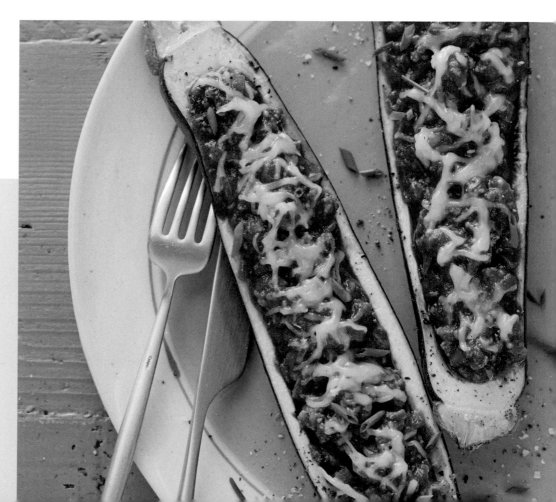

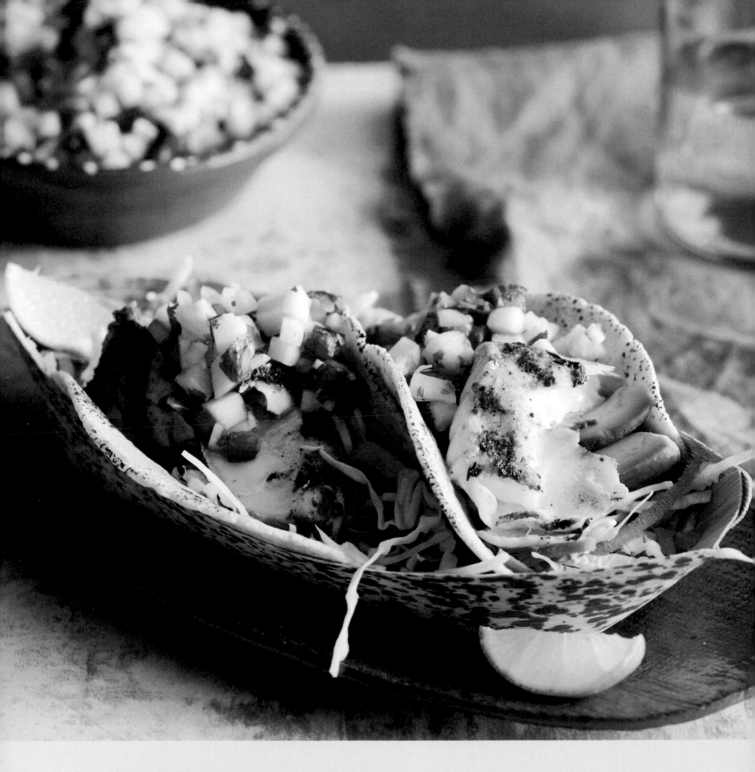

Food as Medicine

Omega-3 fats in fish have been proven to reduce diabetes, heart disease, cancer, and dementia. They lower cholesterol and triglycerides. And they are powerful anti-inflammatory compounds.

Grilled Spicy Fish Tacos

4 (2-ounce) pieces of white fish such as cod or halibut, cut into strips

1 tablespoon coconut oil

2 teaspoons Cajun seasoning

4 organic corn tortillas

½ cup shredded green cabbage

½ cup shredded red cabbage

¼ cup shredded carrots

1 avocado, sliced

½ cup Mango-Jalapeno Salsa

Fish and seafood are great sources of omega-3 fats (as well as protein and minerals). Feel free to use your favorite low-mercury fish for tacos.   **GF** **DF**   **4 tacos**

1. Preheat grill. (You may warm tortillas wrapped in wax paper in a microwave for 15 seconds instead.)

2. Mix Cajun seasoning and oil together. Rub mixture on fish. Grill fish 2 minutes on each side till medium done. Remove from grill. Set aside.

3. Brown tortillas on the grill or warm in microwave.

4. Place a bit of shredded cabbage and carrot on the tortillas. Arrange 2 slices of avocado on top of cabbage. Place grilled fish on avocado, and top with salsa.

Mango-Jalapeno Salsa

1 mango, peeled and diced

½ cup diced pineapple

1 Granny Smith apple, peeled and diced

¼ cup seeded and diced tomato

¼ cup diced red bell pepper

4 tablespoons lime juice

2 tablespoons minced fresh ginger

2 tablespoons minced seeded jalapeno

½ cup chopped fresh cilantro

Switch up your regular salsa for a tropical version when using fish or chicken in Mexican recipes.   **2 cups**

Place salsa ingredients in a bowl. Mix together well. Chill in refrigerator. (Keeps up to 1 week refrigerated.)

Roast Chicken Tacos

8 small organic corn tortillas

2 cups finely shredded green or red cabbage (or dark lettuce leaves)

2 large Roma tomatoes, diced or sliced thinly

2 avocados, cut into thin wedges

2 cups shredded roast chicken breast

2 ounces shredded jalapeno-jack cheese (optional)

Fresh cilantro (optional)

1–2 large limes cut into quarters

½ cup Creamy Chipotle-Lime Sauce (below)

Skip the fast food taco joints and make tastier, healthier tacos at home. Tacos are the perfect use for leftover shredded roast chicken. You could also use thinly sliced steak, small grilled shrimp, even seasoned and cooked ground beef or turkey. Tacos are so versatile! See recipe for roast chicken breast on page 195.   GF **8 tacos**

1. Warm tortillas for about 30 seconds in the microwave wrapped in waxed paper or in an oven-safe tortilla warmer, until they are soft and pliable.

2. Spread each tortilla with 1 tablespoon of sauce. Top with cabbage, tomato, avocado, chicken, cheese, and cilantro. Squeeze lime over the top.

Creamy Chipotle-Lime Sauce

¼ cup plain Greek yogurt

¼ cup organic or vegan mayonnaise

1 tablespoon lime juice

2 pinches kosher or sea salt

Pinch black pepper

1 garlic clove, minced

⅛ teaspoon chipotle or cayenne powder

Make your tacos sing with this fresh spicy sauce. It works well with any taco meat or toppings.   GF **½ cup**

Whisk all ingredients in a small bowl until smooth.

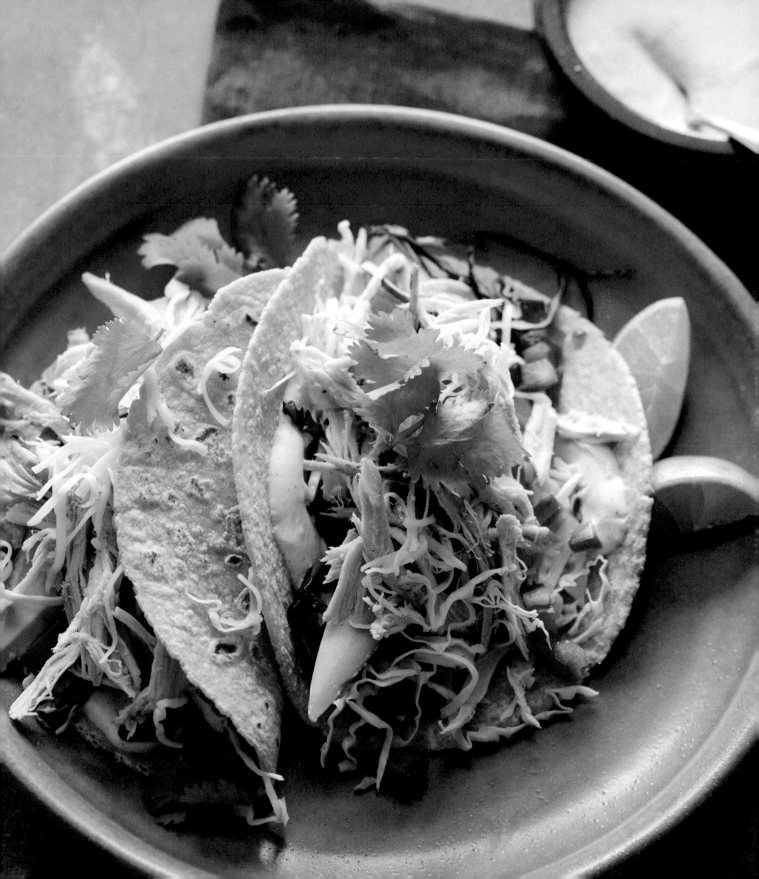

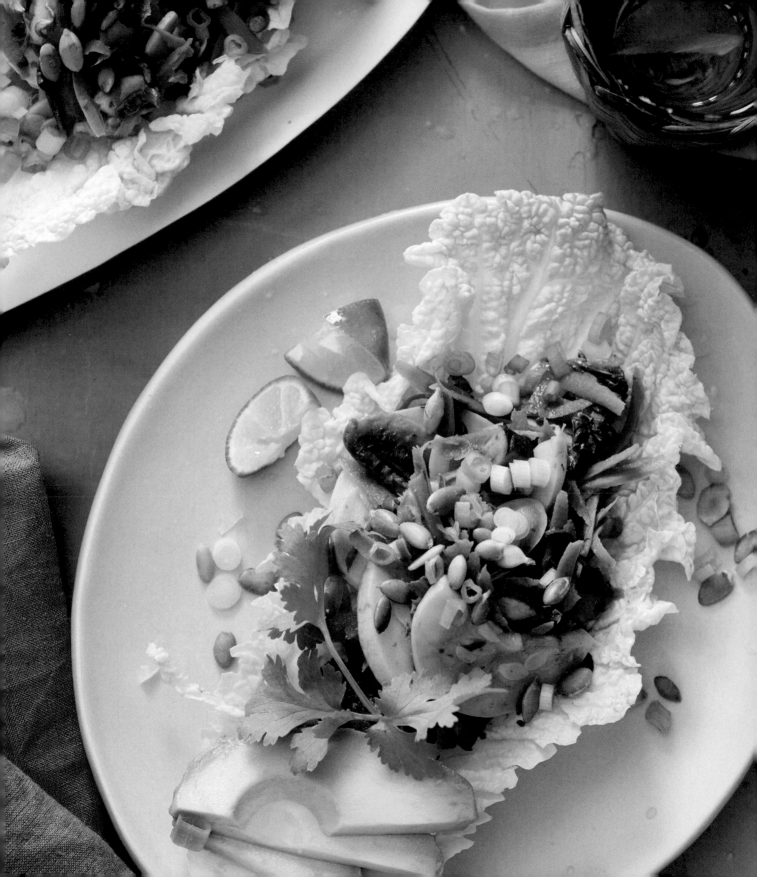

Veggie Tacos

Vegetables

2 cups diced mushrooms

2 cups chopped spinach

2 cups sliced zucchini or yellow crookneck squash

1 cup shredded carrots

Marinade

1 Roma tomato

1 red bell pepper

1 garlic clove

1 green onion

1 dried chipotle pepper

2 tablespoons extra-virgin olive oil

1 teaspoon kosher or sea salt

Tacos

6 organic corn tortillas or small Napa cabbage leaves

1 avocado

⅓ cup chopped green onions

⅓ cup chopped fresh cilantro

Vegetable tacos are a great meatless option for lunch or dinner. These tacos can be made quickly, especially if you prepare the vegetable mix and marinade at the beginning of the week and store it in your refrigerator. Both components also work great in other dishes — as a topping for a salad or sauce for a vegetable sauté.

GF **DF** **V**   6 tacos

1. Toss together mushrooms, spinach, squash, and carrots in a medium mixing bowl. Set aside.

2. Put marinade ingredients into a blender, and puree until smooth. You may benefit from using the immersion blender for small batches of sauce such as this one. It saves time and mess.

3. Steam the vegetable mixture for 5 minutes on the stovetop in a steam pot until the color brightens, and the vegetables begin to soften. Remove from the stove and transfer the vegetable mixture to a mixing bowl.

4. Coat the vegetable mix with ½ cup of the marinade. Toss until all vegetables are well coated. Let sit covered for 5 minutes.

5. Scoop ¾ cup of vegetable mixture into each tortilla or cabbage leaf. Top with diced avocado, green onion, and cilantro. Remaining ingredients will store in the refrigerator for 2 additional days.

> **TIP**   Taco Tuesday in your house can be a fun way to involve the whole family in dinner. Visit a local farm or farmers market each week, and pick out different variations of vegetables for new flavors to try in your tacos. Also check out our Fiesta Party idea on page 256.

Kicking and Screaming
Steak Fajitas

2–4 chipotle peppers in adobo sauce (canned)

½ cup coconut oil

½ cup chopped sweet onion

6 cloves garlic, minced

4 teaspoons lime zest (about 2 limes)

2 teaspoons chili powder

2 teaspoons cumin

2 teaspoons kosher or sea salt

½ teaspoon black pepper

1½ pounds flank steak, trimmed

Extra-virgin olive oil

2 cups sliced bell peppers

1 cup sliced red onion

4–6 organic corn tortillas

½ cup sliced radishes

¼ cup fresh cilantro

1 lime, cut into wedges (use one of the zested limes)

This is a HOT recipe sure to get your blood flowing. Capsaicin, that oil that makes all chiles hot, is great for building red blood cells and equalizing your blood pressure. **GF** **DF** **4–6 servings**

1. Place the chipotle peppers, coconut oil, onion, garlic, zest, spices, salt, and pepper in a blender, and blend until smooth.

2. Place mixture in a gallon-size plastic bag with the flank steak. Let stand on counter 1 hour, turning occasionally, or marinate in the fridge overnight.

3. Remove meat from bag, and wipe off excess marinade.

4. Spray or brush both sides of meat with olive oil. Grill meat over high heat for 3 to 5 minutes on each side until desired doneness. Remove meat from grill and let stand 10 to 15 minutes. Slice the flank steak very thinly across the grain.

5. Grill or sauté bell peppers and onions till tender, about 5 minutes. Set aside, and keep warm.

6. Grill tortillas till warm and flexible. Fill with a few strips of steak, grilled veggies, radishes, and cilantro. Squeeze lime juice over each fajita.

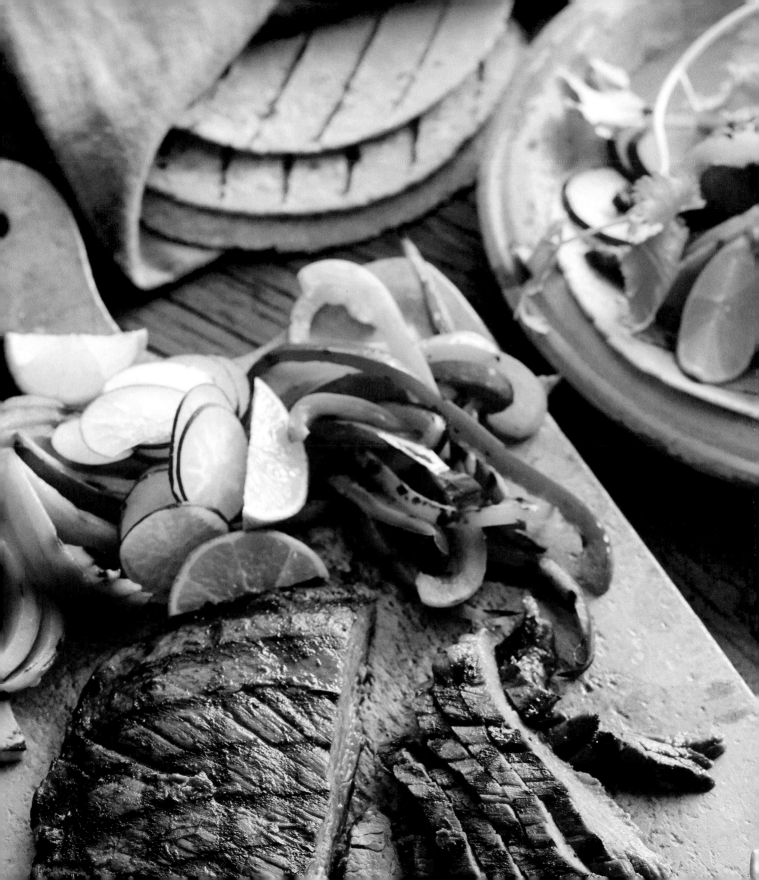

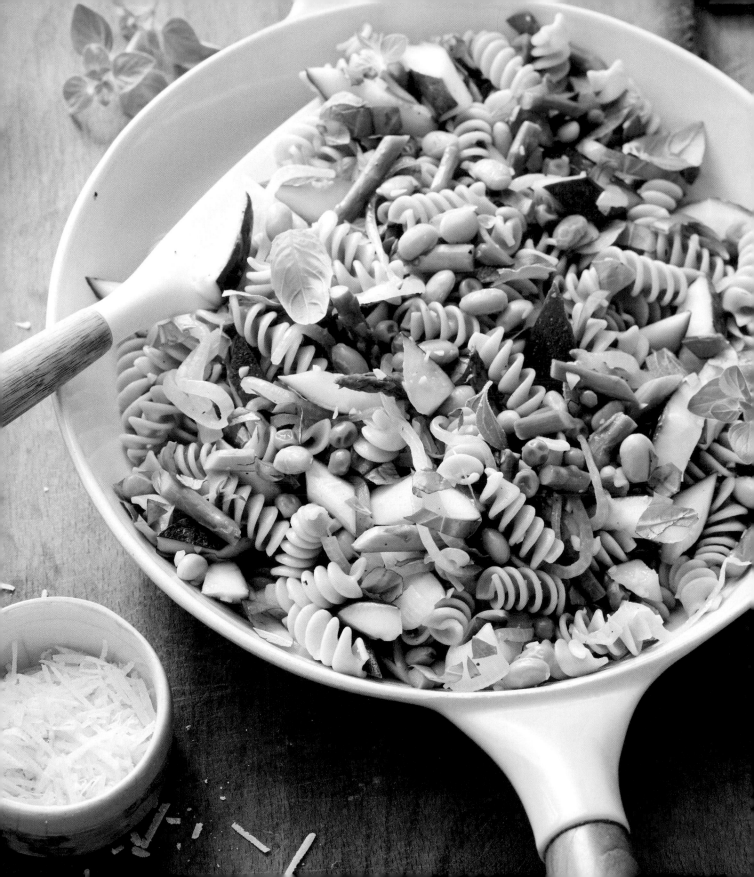

Pasta Primaverde

2–3 teaspoons kosher or sea salt

½ medium onion, thinly sliced

16 medium spears fresh asparagus

3 small zucchini

1½ tablespoons extra-virgin olive oil

1 cup peas (thawed if frozen)

1 cup shelled organic edamame (thawed if frozen)

3–4 large garlic cloves, minced

8 ounces whole wheat or brown rice pasta

4 tablespoons finely chopped fresh herbs (basil, oregano, parsley)

4 tablespoons grated Parmesan cheese (omit for DF)

Black pepper

Skip the creamy, heavy sauce and focus on the fresh clean flavor of green vegetables tossed with pasta and herbs. Cook your pasta shape of preference — spaghetti, farfalle, penne, or linguine. Finish with a sprinkle of a little Parmesan if desired. Use brown rice pasta for a gluten-free dish.

4 servings

1. Fill a large pot three-quarters full (4–5 quarts) of water. Add 2 teaspoons of salt. Bring water to a boil over high heat. While water is coming to a boil, prep your vegetables.

2. Slice onion into thin half rounds. Snap ends off asparagus, then cut on the diagonal into small pieces about ½-inch wide. Trim ends off zucchini and quarter lengthwise. Cut zucchini on the diagonal into small pieces about ½-inch wide.

3. Add the pasta to boiling water and cook according to package directions.

4. In a large sauté pan, heat the olive oil over medium heat. Cook the onion until soft, stirring occasionally. Add peas, asparagus, zucchini, and edamame. Cook until vegetables are crisp-tender when pierced with tip of a sharp knife. Add the garlic, stir and cook 1 minute. Keep vegetables warm until pasta is done.

5. Drain pasta, leaving a little water still clinging to the noodles. Place the drained pasta in the pan with the vegetables. Add herbs. Gently toss together. Drizzle with a little more olive oil, and sprinkle with salt and pepper. Divide pasta and vegetables into wide serving bowls. Sprinkle with cheese if desired.

TIP The best way to control pasta portions (and other ingredients) is to weigh them with a digital kitchen scale, an inexpensive tool and worthwhile investment.

Spaghetti and Meatballs

Meatballs

1 pound ground turkey, beef, buffalo, or lamb

½ cup whole wheat or gluten-free bread crumbs

¼ cup milk or water

1 egg white

¼ cup grated Parmesan cheese

½ teaspoon dried basil

½ teaspoon dried oregano

¼ teaspoon kosher or sea salt

⅛ teaspoon black pepper

2 teaspoons extra-virgin olive oil

Fresh basil (optional garnish)

Spaghetti

8 ounces spaghetti (quinoa, brown rice, multigrain, or whole wheat)

2 quarts water

2 cups organic or Savory Spaghetti Sauce (see page 107)

An American tradition and favorite of kids of all ages! Try this recipe with lean ground turkey, buffalo, or lamb instead of the meatball standard of beef. You might even try combining a few of these into one recipe.

4 servings

1. In a bowl, combine ground turkey with bread crumbs, milk, egg white, cheese, basil, oregano, salt, and pepper. Mix thoroughly. Shape mixture into 12 evenly sized meatballs.

2. Heat olive oil in a large nonstick skillet. Add meatballs and cook over medium heat until meat is no longer pink, turning every so often so meatballs are brown all over, about 5–7 minutes.

3. In a small saucepan, warm spaghetti sauce.

4. In a large pot, bring water to a boil. Add spaghetti. Cook according to package directions, stirring occasionally. Drain. Serve immediately with meatballs and sauce. Garnish with fresh basil if desired.

TIP You'll find many alternatives to white pastas. The Daniel Plan prefers brown rice pasta for its flavor and texture, but we encourage you to experiment with other types made from whole grain, quinoa, shirataki, and buckwheat. Find your favorite, then use it as a substitute for any pasta dish.

Savory Spaghetti Sauce

2 tablespoons extra-virgin olive oil

¼ cup diced celery

¼ cup diced green bell pepper

¼ cup diced red bell pepper

¼ cup diced sweet onions

½ pound tomatoes, diced

3 cloves garlic, minced

1 (28-ounce) can crushed tomatoes

2 tablespoons balsamic vinegar

¼ teaspoon cracked fennel seeds

¼ teaspoon dried basil

¼ teaspoon dried oregano

1 bay leaf

1 teaspoon grated Parmesan cheese (omit for DF/V)

¼ teaspoon black pepper

¼ teaspoon crushed red pepper (omit for mild version)

This recipe is bursting with antioxidants and primo Italian flavors that will make any pasta dish perfect. This also works well for chicken Parmesan, poured over scrambled eggs, or reduced (thickened) for a pizza sauce.

GF **1 quart**

1. Heat olive oil in sauté or frying pan over medium heat.

2. Sauté celery, peppers, and onion till tender, about 5 minutes. Add garlic and tomatoes and cook 1 more minute. Add remaining ingredients, bring to a boil, and simmer for 2 hours.

3. Remove bay leaf. Cool slightly. Place all ingredients in a food processor or blender. Puree until smooth. This sauce keeps for 1 week in the refrigerator.

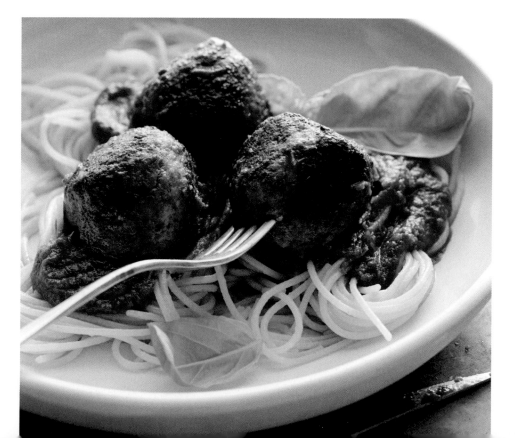

Mac and Cheese

12 ounces brown rice
elbow pasta

3–4 quarts water

1 teaspoon kosher
or sea salt

4 tablespoons grated
Parmesan cheese

4 tablespoons gluten-free
bread crumbs

2 tablespoons plus
2 teaspoons extra-virgin
olive oil

2 cups small cauliflower
florets

½ cup cottage cheese

2¾ cups milk

1 cup chopped onion

3 garlic cloves, minced

¼ teaspoon black pepper

2 tablespoons all-purpose
gluten-free flour

1 generous tablespoon
Dijon mustard

4 ounces shredded extra
sharp cheddar cheese

2 ounces grated Parmesan
cheese

Classic macaroni and cheese gets an update with cauliflower puree and rice pasta for a gluten-free comfort food dish. Add a big tossed green or chopped vegetable salad for a balanced plate.

GF 6 servings

1. Fill a large pot ¾ full with water. Bring water to a boil and add ½ teaspoon of the salt. Cook pasta according to package directions. Drain well and toss with 1 teaspoon of the olive oil to prevent sticking.

2. While pasta is cooking, lightly oil a 9 × 13 baking dish.

3. Combine Parmesan, bread crumbs, and remaining 1 teaspoon of oil. Toss with a fork to combine.

4. Pre-heat oven 350˚.

5. Steam cauliflower for 12–15 minutes until very soft. Drain and place in the bowl of a food processor. Puree cauliflower with cottage cheese and only ½ cup milk until smooth.

6. Heat 1 tablespoon olive oil in a sauté pan over medium-low heat. Add onion, and cook until soft but not browned, about 7–8 minutes. Add garlic and cook 1 minute. Add the remaining ½ teaspoon of the salt and ¼ teaspoon pepper.

7. Add 1 more tablespoon olive oil and flour. Cook flour and onion mixture for 2–3 minutes until thickened. Add the remaining milk and stir or whisk until smooth and thickened. Add the mustard and cheeses. Continue to stir or whisk until cheese is melted and sauce is smooth. Add the cauliflower puree to the pan, and stir to combine.

8. Combine cooked pasta and sauce in a large bowl and stir to coat well. Pour into baking dish. Evenly sprinkle the crumb topping over the top of the pasta. Bake uncovered for approximately 30 minutes or until the top has a golden crust. Allow to stand for a few minutes, then serve.

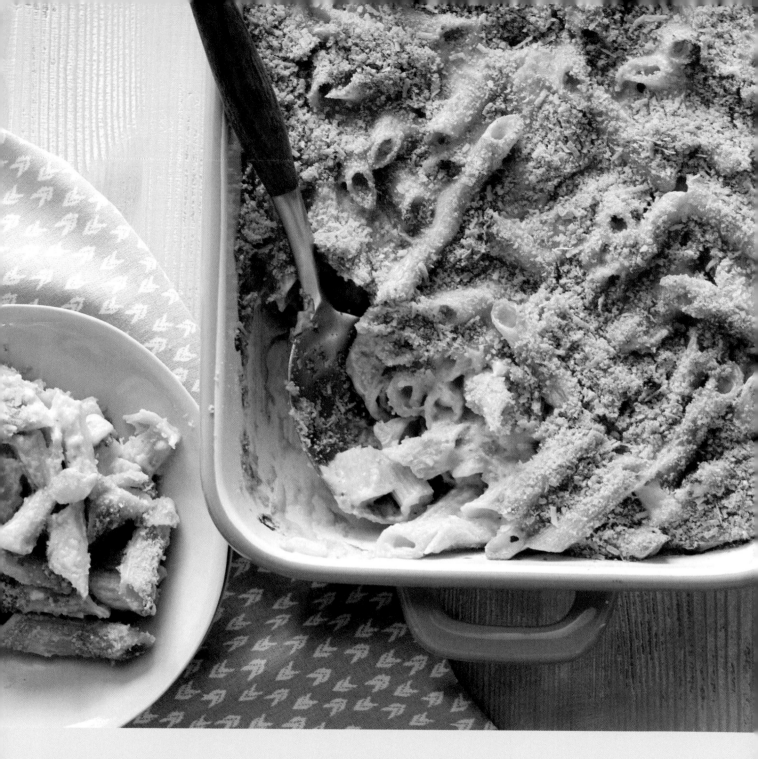

Food as Medicine

The one variety you can never get enough of is the cruciferous vegetable family, which includes kale, collards, broccoli, cabbage, Brussels sprouts, cauliflower, and bok choy. They contain powerful detoxifying chemicals called glucosinolates that prevent cancer and support your health.

Five-Veggie Lasagna

Topping Sauce

1½ cups cubed butternut squash

1 cup water

2 Roma tomatoes

2 cloves garlic

1 teaspoon kosher or sea salt

4 tablespoons Italian seasoning

3 tablespoons extra-virgin olive oil

Creamy Sauce

2 cups macadamia nuts

1 cup water

2 Roma tomatoes

⅔ cup lemon juice

1 tablespoon kosher or sea salt

1½ cups chopped cauliflower

4 cups chopped spinach

Filling

4 cups diced eggplant or yellow crookneck squash

4 cups diced tomato

4 cups corn

Noodle Layer

6 zucchini or yellow crookneck squash or 8 large brown rice lasagna noodles

Extra-virgin olive oil

Vegetables are the highlight of this lasagna, creating a new twist on a classic dish, except this version is nutrient rich and Daniel Plan–approved! The five-vegetable lasagna is a layered dish with three key parts: filling, creamy sauce, and topping. If you prepare each section separately and then focus on assembly, you will have this dish done in no time. **GF DF V 6–8 servings**

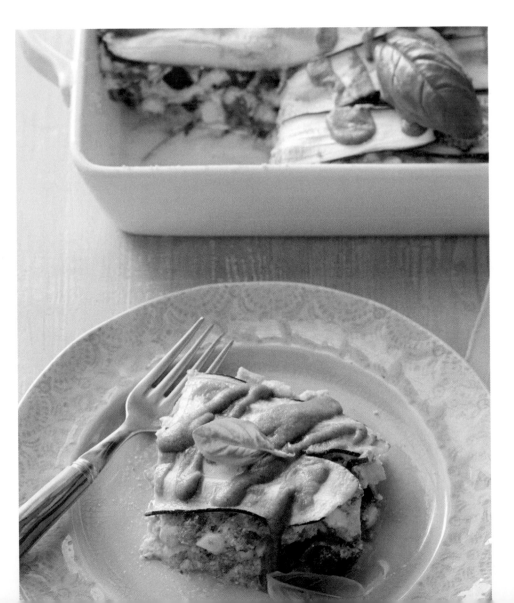

TIP Use the creamy sauce as a dip or a spread on other dishes. The topping doubles as a hidden gem for spaghetti and other pasta dishes. Make two batches so you have one for later.

1. Blend the butternut squash, water, tomatoes, garlic, salt, and Italian seasoning for the topping in a blender until a vegetable puree has formed. Add the olive oil and turn the blender back on to help create a creamy rich vegetable mixture. Pour the mixture into a separate bowl or container and set aside. Store this sauce for up to 3 days in the refrigerator; stir prior to use.

2. In the same blender, blend the macadamia nuts, water, tomatoes, lemon juice, salt, and cauliflower until a rich creamy sauce has formed. Pour the mixture into a separate bowl, and fold in the spinach. Set aside this mixture. This mixture will also save for up to 3 days in the refrigerator.

3. In a medium mixing bowl, toss together the eggplant, tomato, and corn with 3 tablespoons of the topping, and let sit while preparing the noodles.

4. If making squash "noodles," use a mandoline slicing tool to slice the squash, after removing the stem and the bottom ¼ inch of the squash. Move the squash lengthwise over the mandoline set at ⅛-inch. Each squash is different so you may need to make some basic adjustments for the number of slices necessary to create a layer. For the brown rice pasta version, prepare the noodles according to the package directions.

5. Preheat oven to 350°.

6. Lightly oil a 9 × 13 lasagna pan. Place half of the vegetable mixture evenly in the pan, then arrange a layer of noodles, top with half of the creamy sauce then 4 tablespoons of the topping sauce. Repeat.

7. Finish by adding one final layer of noodles on the very top of the dish. Pour the remaining topping over the top. This will fill your baking pan to the top. As the mixture cooks, it will condense and set up perfectly.

8. Bake the lasagna for 25 minutes. Remove from the oven, and let cool. Cut into 6 equal portions. Extra portions will keep refrigerated for up to 3 days.

9. If you are using the squash noodles, you will notice some liquid has collected in your pan. This is a natural process as the squash expels moisture in the cooking process. After letting cool, gently tip your lasagna tray over the sink to pour off the extra moisture.

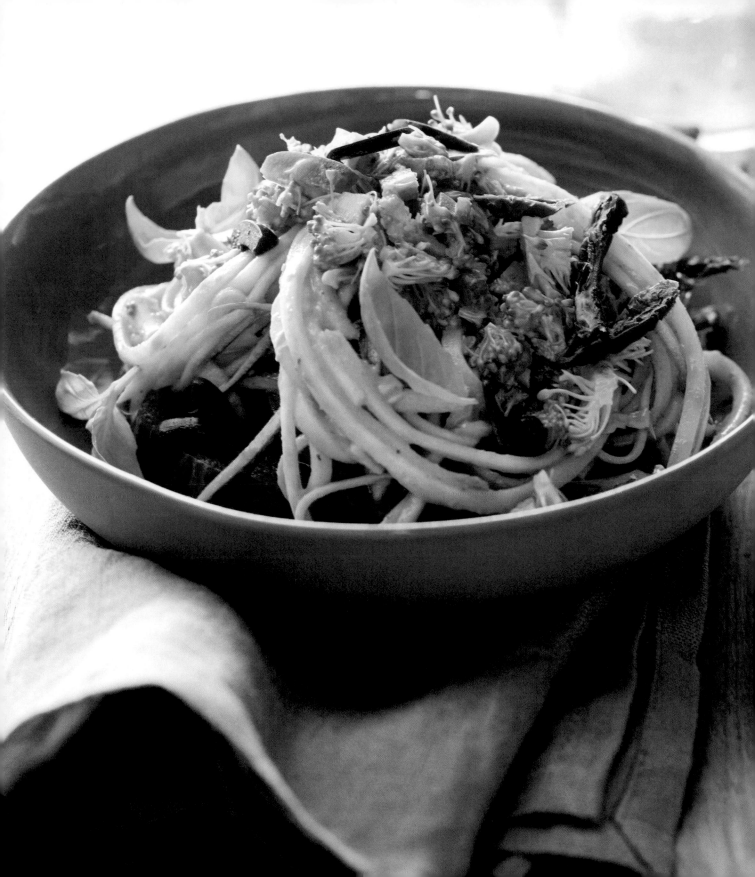

Zucchini Pasta

Pasta

2 medium zucchini

Sauce

½ cup water

1 tablespoon raw honey

2 Roma tomatoes, roughly chopped

2 sun-dried tomatoes

1 red bell pepper

⅓ cup fresh basil leaves

3 tablespoons extra-virgin olive oil

1 teaspoon kosher or sea salt

Topping

¼ cup Kalamata olives, pitted and chopped

½ cup diced Roma tomatoes

½ cup finely chopped broccoli or red bell peppers

4 tablespoons grated Parmesan cheese (omit for DF)

Noodles can be a high quality meal when made from zucchini! Full of fiber, vitamins, and minerals, and naturally hydrating, zucchini make a great stand-in for more traditional pastas. Use this recipe as a base for your next pasta bar or as a Daniel Plan alternative at your next dinner party or potluck. This dish works nicely as a stand-alone entrée but also makes a great side dish for fish and chicken.

GF DF V **2–4 servings**

1. With a mandoline, vegetable peeler, or a vegetable spiralizer, thinly slice zucchini into long julienne strips to form thin "noodles." A mandoline set on the julienne blade is the easiest tool to use for this. Put the noodles in a large mixing bowl then set aside.

2. Combine all sauce ingredients in a blender (liquids first makes for an easier blend), and blend on high until smooth.

3. Pour the sauce over the noodles, and toss well until evenly coated. Top each serving with even portions of the toppings, and enjoy immediately.

Optional: Prepare the noodles, sauce, and toppings in advance and store separately in the refrigerator for up to 5 days. Then for best results, when you are ready to enjoy, leave the items out until they warm to room temperature.

TIP If you plan to purchase a mandolin for easy, quick vegetable slicing, look for one with sturdy grips on the bottom and a rotating blade. The device also comes with a guard to protect your fingers. One trick is to purchase a gardening glove, and wear it when using a mandolin so you can get the most pieces out of each vegetable.

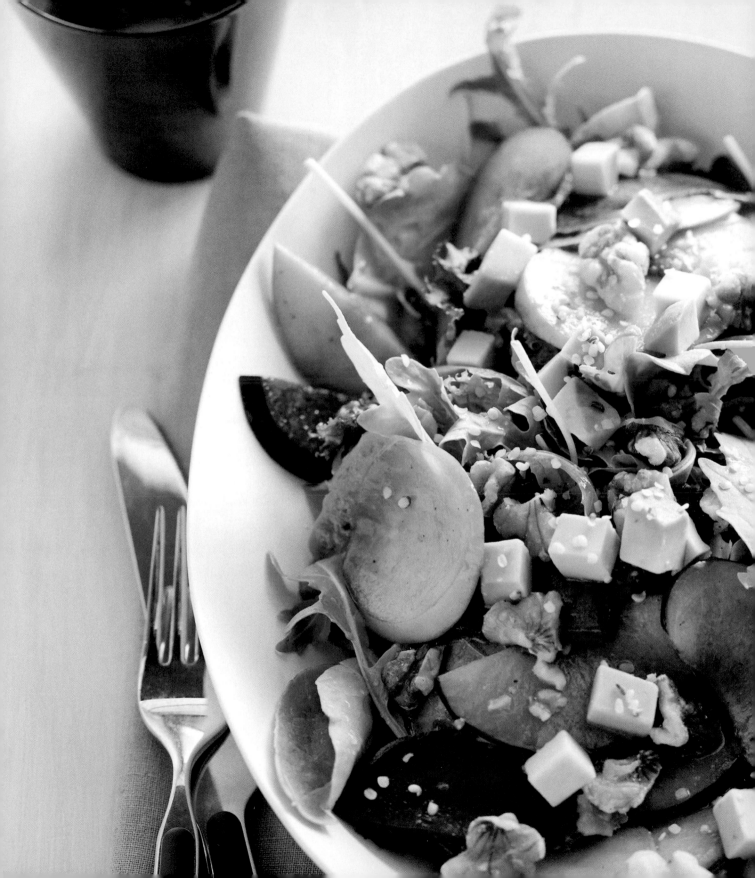

Salads, Sandwiches, and Wraps

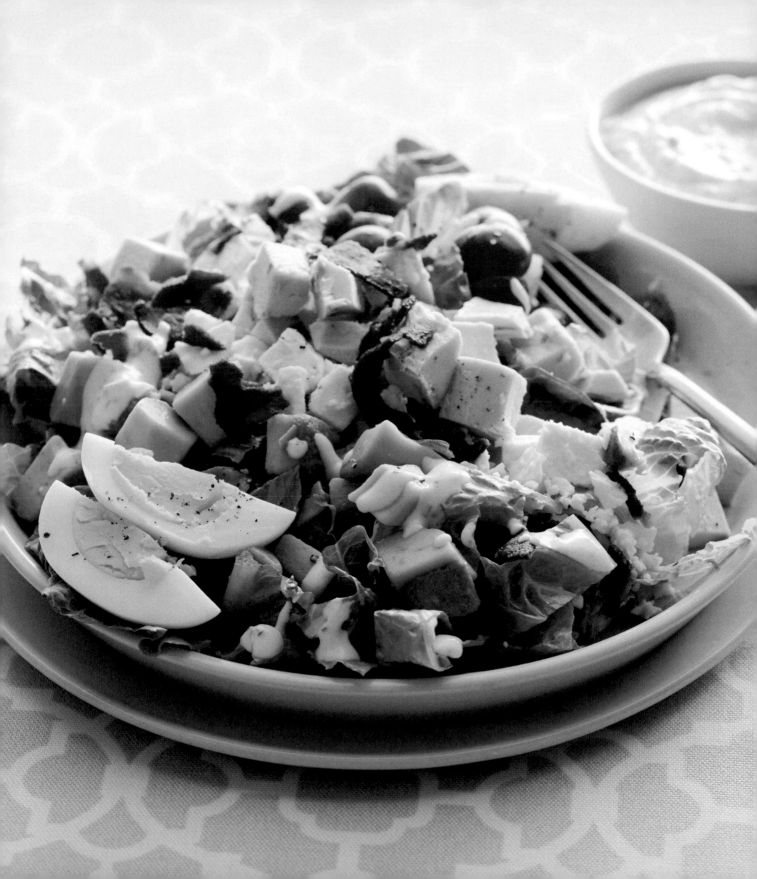

Cobb Salad

1 small grilled or baked chicken breast

1 head romaine lettuce, chopped

1 cup grape tomatoes, sliced in half

1 avocado, diced

4 hard-boiled eggs, cut into quarters

8 pieces turkey bacon, cooked crispy and crumbled

4 ounces crumbled feta cheese

Homemade Ranch Dressing (below)

The Cobb salad is an American main dish. Try this Daniel Plan version with lean turkey bacon and feta cheese.   **GF   4 servings**

1. Dice chicken breast into ½-inch cubes.

2. Divide the lettuce onto 4 plates, then top with the chicken, tomatoes, feta, and avocado. Sprinkle bacon crumbles onto each salad.

3. Drizzle ranch dressing over salad. Place egg wedges on the outer rim of each plate.

Homemade Ranch Dressing

½ cup organic or vegan mayonnaise

2 tablespoons water

1 tablespoon lemon juice

2 cloves garlic, minced

1 tablespoon minced fresh basil

½ teaspoon minced chives

Kosher or sea salt

Black pepper

Besides ketchup, ranch dressing is about as American as it gets. Make your own to ensure good-for-you ingredients, then use it on salads, sandwiches, fries, and pizza crusts.   **GF   4 servings**

1. Combine all ingredients in a small bowl. Whisk well.

2. Refrigerate 15 minutes. Make this dressing ahead of time, and store it in the refrigerator for about a week.

Tangy Chicken Caesar Salad

Dressing

6 ounces plain Greek yogurt

¼ cup organic or vegan mayonnaise

1 tablespoon lemon juice

1 tablespoon Dijon mustard

2–3 teaspoons Worcestershire sauce (without HFCS)

2 tablespoons extra-virgin olive oil

1 large garlic clove, crushed

2 teaspoons white wine or champagne vinegar

1–2 tablespoons milk (optional)

Quick Chicken Breast

1–1 ½ pounds boneless, skinless chicken breast

Kosher or sea salt, black pepper, and granulated garlic powder

1 tablespoon extra-virgin olive oil

¾ cup chicken broth

Salad

Romaine lettuce

2–3 tablespoons finely chopped red onion or shallot (optional)

4–6 tablespoons cooked corn (optional)

4 teaspoons chopped fresh parsley

4 tablespoons grated Parmesan cheese

The classic flavors of a Caesar salad start with the creamy dressing, but typically the store-bought versions are filled with unhealthy additives. The Daniel Plan version has full flavor, healthy ingredients, and a few colorful additions. **GF** **4 servings**

1. Whisk all ingredients for the dressing together in a medium bowl. Thin with a little extra milk to desired consistency. Set aside in the refrigerator.

2. Sprinkle chicken breasts with salt, pepper, and granulated garlic. Heat oil over medium heat in a sauté pan. Place the chicken breasts top side (smooth side) down and cook until golden, 3–4 minutes.

3. Turn chicken over, pour in broth, and immediately cover with a lid. Turn heat to low. Allow chicken to finish cooking, until the chicken breast is firm and internal temperature reads 160°–165° with a digital thermometer.

4. Trim the bottom of the head of Romaine, then separate leaves onto plates, or chop leaves crosswise into strips.

5. Slice the chicken, and divide into four portions. Place chicken slices on lettuce. Sprinkle with red onion, corn, parsley, and Parmesan. Serve dressing on the side.

TIP For many people, a great Caesar Salad isn't the same without croutons. For gluten-free croutons, trim crusts from gluten-free bread, cut into large cubes, toss with a little olive oil, garlic powder, salt, and pepper and bake at 300° until golden, dry, and crunchy. Cool and add to salad.

BLT Steak Salad

½ teaspoon kosher or sea salt

½ teaspoon granulated garlic powder

½ teaspoon onion powder

½ teaspoon paprika

¼ teaspoon black pepper

1-pound flank steak, trimmed

2 tablespoons extra-virgin olive oil, plus extra for greasing

2 tablespoons red wine vinegar

1 tablespoon organic or vegan mayonnaise

1 teaspoon Dijon mustard

1 teaspoon Italian seasoning

6 cups romaine lettuce, cut into bite-size pieces

1 cup grape tomatoes, cut in half

1 red onion, diced

¼ cup crumbled blue cheese

4 slices turkey bacon, cooked crispy and crumbled

Everyone loves a BLT. Turn it into a hearty salad and serve it as an entrée to please a crowd. 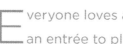 **4 servings**

1. Mix ¼ teaspoon of the salt, garlic, onion, paprika, and pepper together. Sprinkle on the steak.

2. Fire up the grill, and cook till desired doneness, or heat a nonstick grill pan with olive oil over medium-high heat. Add the steak, and cook 5 minutes on each side for medium rare. Transfer the steak to a cutting board, and let rest 5 minutes.

3. Cut the steak on an angle against the grain into 12 slices.

4. Whisk together the oil, vinegar, mayonnaise, mustard, Italian seasoning, and remaining ¼ teaspoon salt in a large bowl. Add the lettuce, tomatoes, and onions. Toss to coat well. Transfer the salad to a platter. Top with the steak slices, and sprinkle with the blue cheese and turkey bacon.

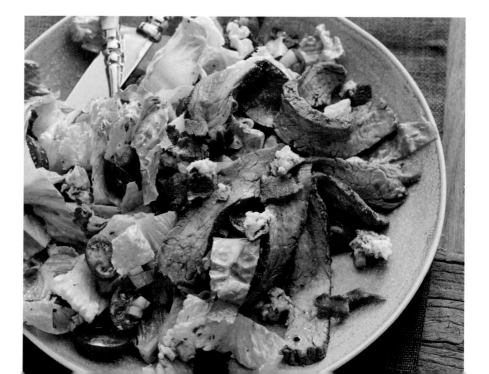

Chinese Chicken Salad

2 hearts of romaine, washed and dried

½ head Napa cabbage, washed and dried

¼–½ small head purple cabbage (optional)

1–1¼ pounds cooked, sliced, or shredded chicken breast (page 195)

4 tablespoons slivered almonds

4 tablespoons sliced green onions

1 large carrot, finely grated or shredded

1 can (11-ounce) mandarin orange segments in water

4 ounces snow peas, cooked and sliced crosswise

2 tablespoons minced fresh cilantro or Italian parsley (optional)

This colorful, refreshing salad is easy to make with leftover chicken breast and canned mandarin orange segments. Almonds add crunch. Purple cabbage, carrot, green onions, and cilantro add color, and the creamy dressing really punches up the flavor! Everything can be done ahead then assembled when ready. **GF** **DF** **4 servings**

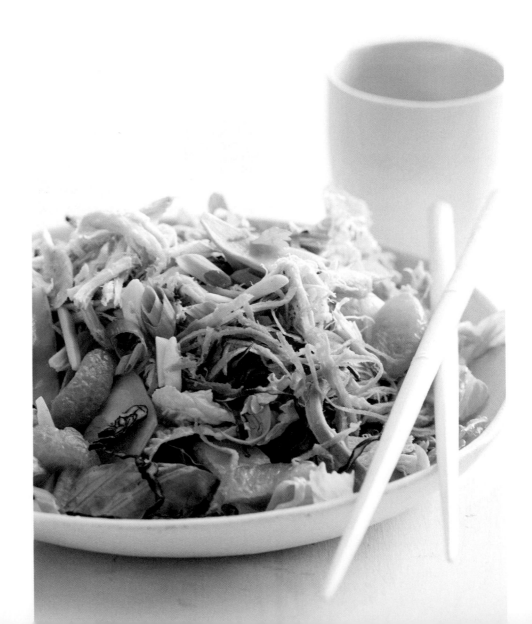

1. Chop romaine crosswise into thin strips. Trim the v-shaped core out of the Napa cabbage. Chop remaining leaves crosswise. Thinly slice or grate the purple cabbage.

2. Divide greens and cabbage onto 4 plates. Arrange the chicken on top of greens, then sprinkle with almonds, green onions, carrot, orange segments, snow peas, and cilantro. Serve dressing on the side.

> **TIP**   Substitute asparagus spears for the snow peas. Cut on the diagonal into approximately ½-inch pieces. Drop into boiling, salted water for 2 minutes, drain, and place in a bowl of ice water to stop the cooking process and chill.

Creamy Ginger-Orange Dressing

3 tablespoons coconut or avocado oil

4 tablespoons orange juice

1 tablespoon wheat-free tamari or soy sauce

1 tablespoon unseasoned rice vinegar or white wine vinegar

2–3 teaspoons finely grated ginger

1 teaspoon toasted sesame oil

1 tablespoon almond butter

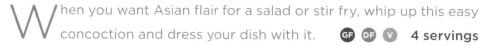

When you want Asian flair for a salad or stir fry, whip up this easy concoction and dress your dish with it.   **GF** **DF** **V**   **4 servings**

1. Place all ingredients in a blender, and puree until smooth. An immersion blender works better for blending small amounts of liquid. You may also put the ingredients in a small sealable container and vigorously shake it to combine.

2. Store in the refrigerator for up to 5 days.

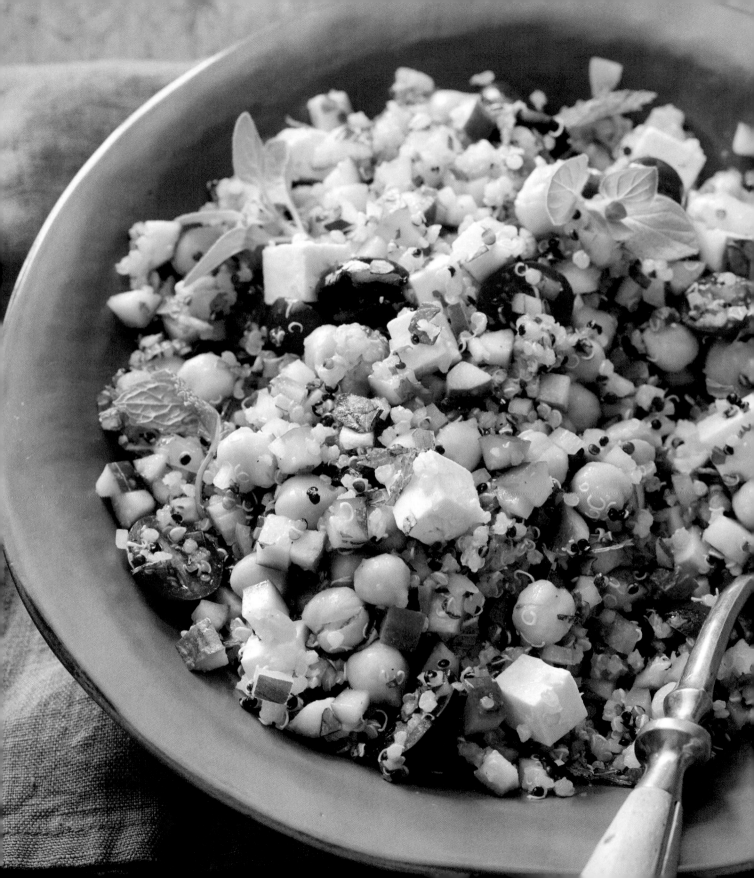

Mediterranean Quinoa Salad

1 cup uncooked quinoa (red, white or tri-color blend)

2 cups water

3 mini cucumbers or 1 English cucumber

12–15 pitted Kalamata olives

½ small red onion, finely chopped

3–4 ounces crumbled feta cheese

18 grape or cherry tomatoes, cut in half

1 yellow bell pepper, finely chopped

¼ cup minced fresh mint leaves

2 tablespoons minced fresh oregano leaves

1 (15-ounce) can garbanzo beans, rinsed and drained

Vinaigrette

5 tablespoons extra-virgin olive oil

3 tablespoons lemon juice

Kosher or sea salt and black pepper

1–2 garlic cloves, minced

Quinoa, the ancient high-protein, gluten-free grain (really a seed) of the Inca Indians, makes a hearty base for this salad. Add lots of colorful vegetables, a little feta, fresh herbs, and an olive oil vinaigrette.

GF **4–6 servings**

1. Place quinoa in a sieve, and rinse well under cold running water for a few minutes. Place rinsed quinoa in a small (2-quart) pan, and add 2 cups water. Bring to a boil. Cover pan with a tight-fitting lid and turn heat to low. Cook quinoa for 18 minutes. Move the pan off the hot burner, and allow to sit for about 7 minutes. Fluff the quinoa with a fork and turn out onto a large, flat, rimmed baking sheet, waxed paper, or foil. Allow quinoa to cool. The larger the surface area, the faster it will cool.

2. While quinoa is cooking or cooling, prep vegetables. Quarter cucumbers lengthwise. Cut quarters into halves, and then chop finely crosswise. Halve the olives. Chop the onion. Cut the feta into very small cubes. Halve the tomatoes. Finely chop the bell pepper.

3. When quinoa is cool, place in a large bowl. Add the vegetables and cheese; mix gently. Serve dressing on the side. Extra dressing will keep a few days in the refrigerator for use over salads or for drizzling over vegetables.

> **TIP** Quinoa must be rinsed because of a natural outer bitter coating called saponin. Cooked quinoa freezes well, so make a large batch to save time in the kitchen for other recipes.
>
> **GOAT'S MILK** is more easily digestible than cow's milk for many people. Look for goat milk cheeses as an alternative.

Mixed Berry Salad

Sweet Berry Dressing

1 cup hulled strawberries

½ cup extra-virgin olive oil

2 drops liquid stevia extract

1 teaspoon kosher or sea salt

Salad

8 cups mixed greens

2 cups fresh mixed berries

2 cups julienned cucumber

1 avocado, diced (optional)

Berries are low-glycemic fruit, important for delivering nutrients that benefit every major system of the body. Use whichever berries you love for this salad, but the contrast of blackberries and strawberries is particularly enjoyable. **GF** **DF** **V** **2–4 servings**

1. Blend strawberries, oil, stevia, and salt in a blender until the mixture is smooth. This dressing will keep up to 5 days in the refrigerator.

2. In a medium bowl, toss together berries, mixed greens, and diced avocado with 1 cup of dressing until well coated. Top with equal parts of the cucumber.

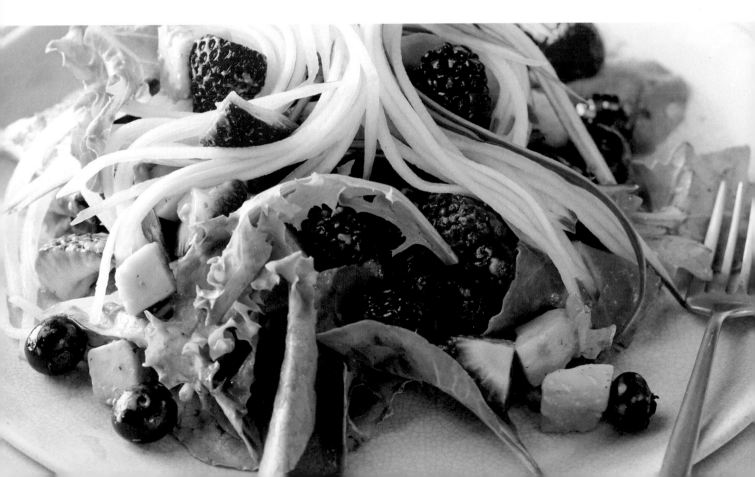

Stone Fruit Salad

Dressing

⅓ cup balsamic vinegar

1 cup extra-virgin olive oil

2 drops liquid stevia extract

1 teaspoon kosher or sea salt

2 tablespoons dried Italian seasoning

Salad

2 cups baby arugula

4 cups mixed greens

2 cups thinly sliced mixed stone fruit

1 avocado, diced

4 tablespoons walnut pieces

Stone fruit includes peaches, nectarines, plums, and cherries as well as special varieties like dino-eggs and sweet saturns. Stone fruit creates a lovely sweet salad for the summer. You'll find stone fruit in any basic grocery store, but they are especially flavorful from the farmers market or picked fresh. **GF** **DF** **V** **2–4 servings**

1. Blend the vinegar, oil, stevia, salt, and Italian seasoning in a blender until smooth. Dressing will keep in the refrigerator for up to 10 days.

2. Gently clean the greens, dry them out completely, then toss them together.

3. In a small mixing bowl, toss the stone fruit slices with 2 tablespoons of the dressing.

4. Plate the greens. Arrange the stone fruit over the top of the greens. Top with diced avocado. Sprinkle with walnut pieces.

Kale Salad

Mustard Dressing

1 cup diced red bell pepper

½ cup extra-virgin olive oil

¼ cup lemon juice

1 tablespoon white miso paste or sea salt

1 clove garlic, minced

Salad

8 cups finely chopped kale

1 avocado, diced

½ cup grape or cherry tomatoes, sliced in half

2 cups julienned or diced cucumber

⅔ cup walnut pieces

If you are new to kale, this salad will make you a fan. It is slightly sweet to offset the naturally bitter elements of the kale and has a great crunchy texture. Kale can be an important staple in any Daniel Plan kitchen. **GF** **DF** **2–4 servings**

1. Put bell papper, olive oil, lemon juice, miso, and garlic in a blender, and puree until smooth. Set aside.

2. In a medium bowl, combine the kale, avocado, cucumber, and walnuts. Using a spatula, fold together the salad ingredients until the avocado naturally starts to coat the kale.

3. Add the tomatoes and salad dressing. Toss together until the salad is coated with dressing and all ingredients are combined, creating a colorful medley.

Food as Medicine

Kale is part of the cabbage family and is at the top of the charts for nutrition density per bite. One cup of chopped kale contains 33 calories and 9% of the daily value of calcium, 206% of vitamin A, 134% of vitamin C, and a whopping 684% of vitamin K. It is also a good source of minerals copper, potassium, iron, manganese, and phosphorus.

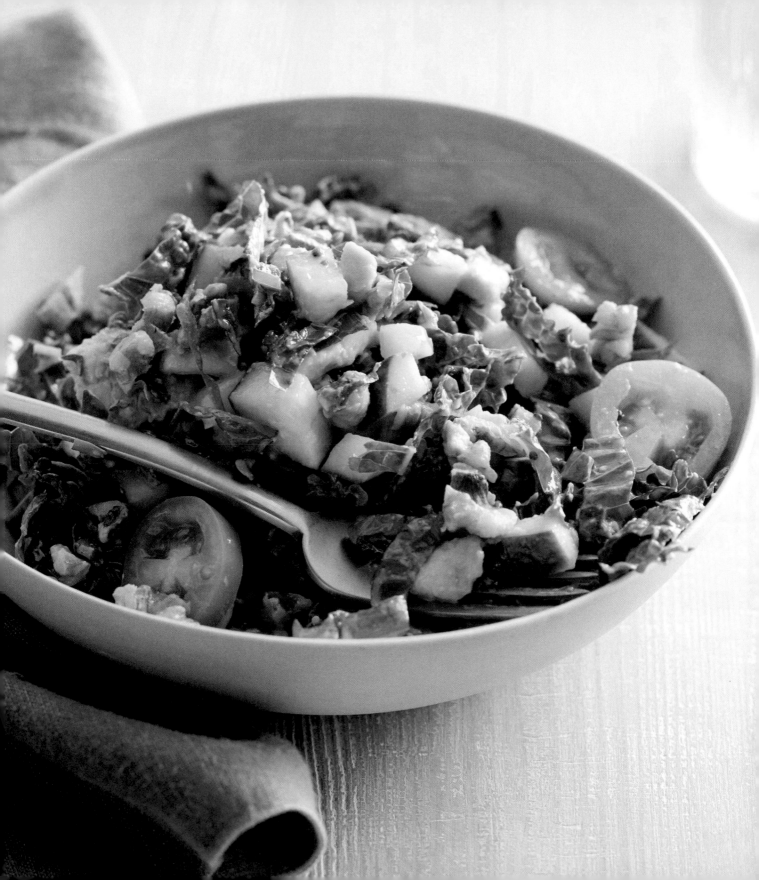

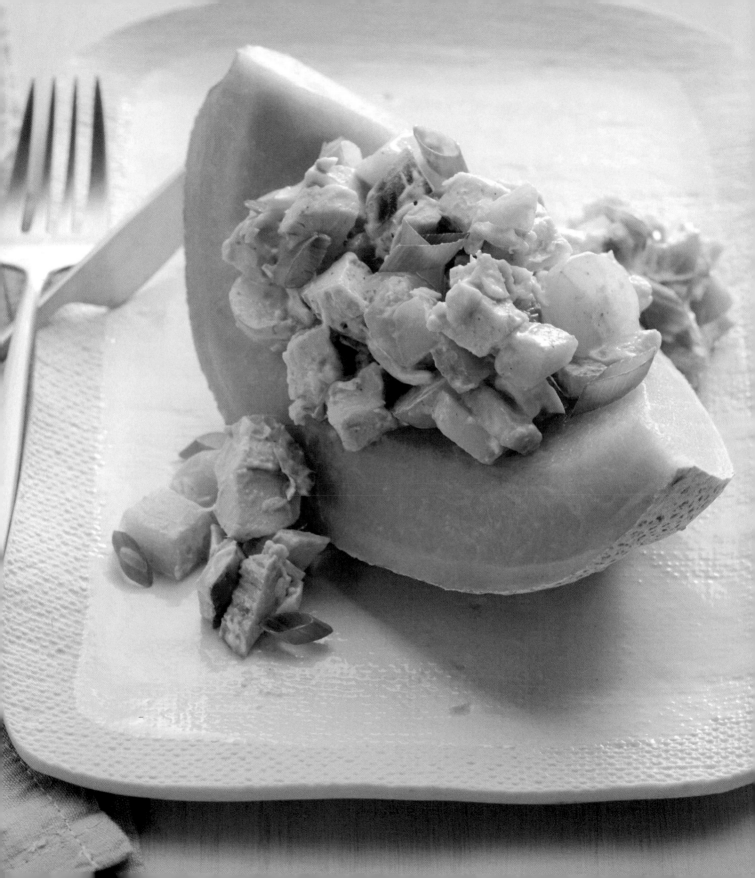

Curried Chicken Salad and Melon

½ cup organic or vegan mayonnaise

1 tablespoon curry powder

2 chicken breasts, boiled and shredded

1 large peach, diced

1 large green onion, chopped

8–10 green grapes, cut in half

½ teaspoon kosher or sea salt

1 medium cantaloupe, seeded and halved

Pastor Warren Family Favorite

Curry powder is a mixture of any number of pungent Indian spices. Yellow curry powder is the most common curry in the U.S., but feel free to change up this recipe with any curry powder that you enjoy.

GF **DF**   **2 servings**

1. In a medium bowl, whisk together mayonnaise and curry powder until smooth.

2. Gently fold shredded chicken, peaches, green onions, grapes, and salt into the curry mixture.

3. Halve the cantaloupes, and discard seeds. Divide the chicken mixture evenly between the two halves of the cantaloupe, and serve cold.

Food as Medicine

One peach is only 37 calories on average, making the peach a low-calorie source of B vitamins, vitamin K, which is essential for healthy blood, and vitamin E, which promotes healthy hair, skin, and nails.

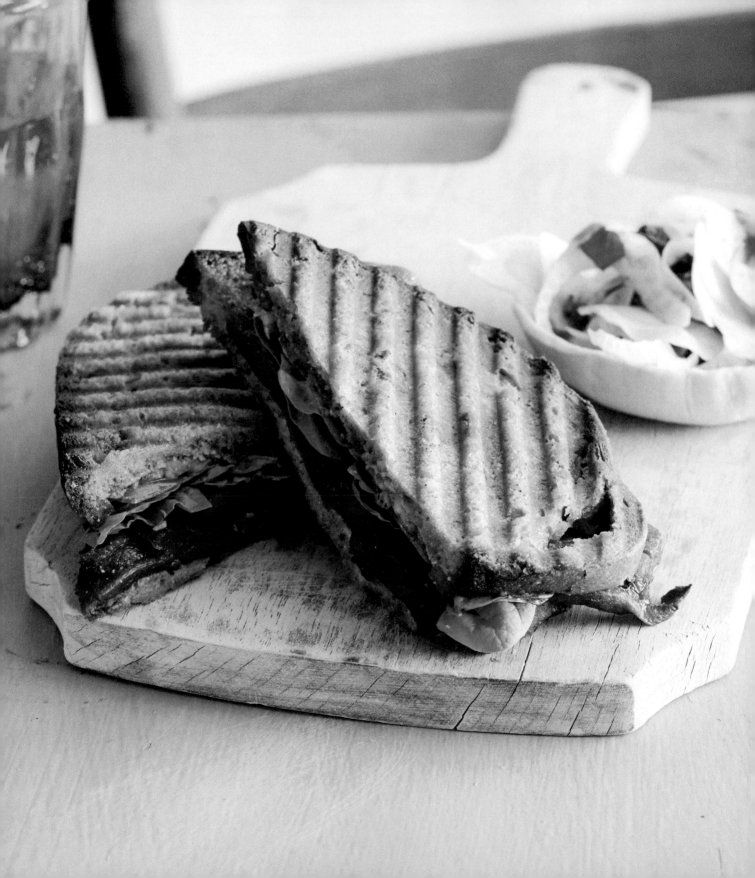

Gluten-Free Pesto Panini

Pesto

1 cup fresh basil leaves

1 cup extra-virgin olive oil

4 cloves garlic

1 teaspoon kosher
or sea salt

½ cup raw pistachios

Panini

4 slices gluten-free bread

2–4 tablespoons oil (your choice)

2 Roma tomatoes, thinly sliced

12 spinach leaves

4 marinated red bell peppers

When transitioning your diet, it may feel like old favorites are not an option, but by simply changing a few ingredients, you'll find new versions that taste great and are still satisfying!

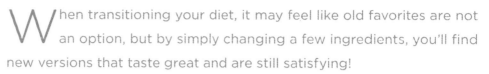 **GF** **DF** **V**   **2 servings**

1. Blend basil, olive oil, garlic, and salt in a food processor until smooth. Add pistachios, and blend until a thick pesto has formed. Remove the pesto from the blender, and store in an airtight container in the refrigerator. This pesto will keep for 7–10 days.

2. Spread oil on one side of each slice of bread. One easy way to accomplish this is to mist the bread with a basic oil sprayer that you can refill with your own oil.

3. Spread the other sides of the bread slices with 1½ tablespoons of pesto. Top one side with tomato, spinach, and red bell pepper. Place the second slice over the top, press down lightly to secure all ingredients in place. Repeat for each sandwich.

4. Heat a skillet over medium heat, and place the sandwich into the skillet. Let warm for 1 minute, then press down on the sandwich with a sandwich press or a spatula. After the bread has crisped on the outside, flip over and repeat.

Food as Medicine

This pesto is anti-inflammatory, anti-bacterial, and a great source of magnesium! Garlic and basil are powerful immune boosters, and this pesto is dairy free. Use it also as a salad dressing, dip, or marinade.

Lemony Dill
Chicken Salad Pita

3 cups chopped cooked
chicken breast

4 small celery ribs, finely
chopped

4 tablespoons finely
chopped red onion

1 generous tablespoon
fresh dill, minced

4 tablespoons organic or
vegan mayonnaise

2 teaspoons lemon juice

Kosher or sea salt and
black pepper (or lemon
pepper)

2 large whole wheat pitas,
sliced in half

Red lettuce leaves

Sliced tomato (optional)

Enjoy a slight twist on a classic chicken salad. For more lemon fla-vor, use the zest too. If dill is not your favorite herb, swap it out for fresh thyme or mint. Why not try this also as an open-face sandwich on gluten-free bread or rolled into a brown rice tortilla?

DF   **4 servings**

1. In a medium bowl, gently mix chicken, celery, onion, mayonnaise, dill, lemon juice, salt, and pepper.

2. Fill each pita half with a lettuce leaf, a slice or two of tomato, then a quarter of the chicken salad.

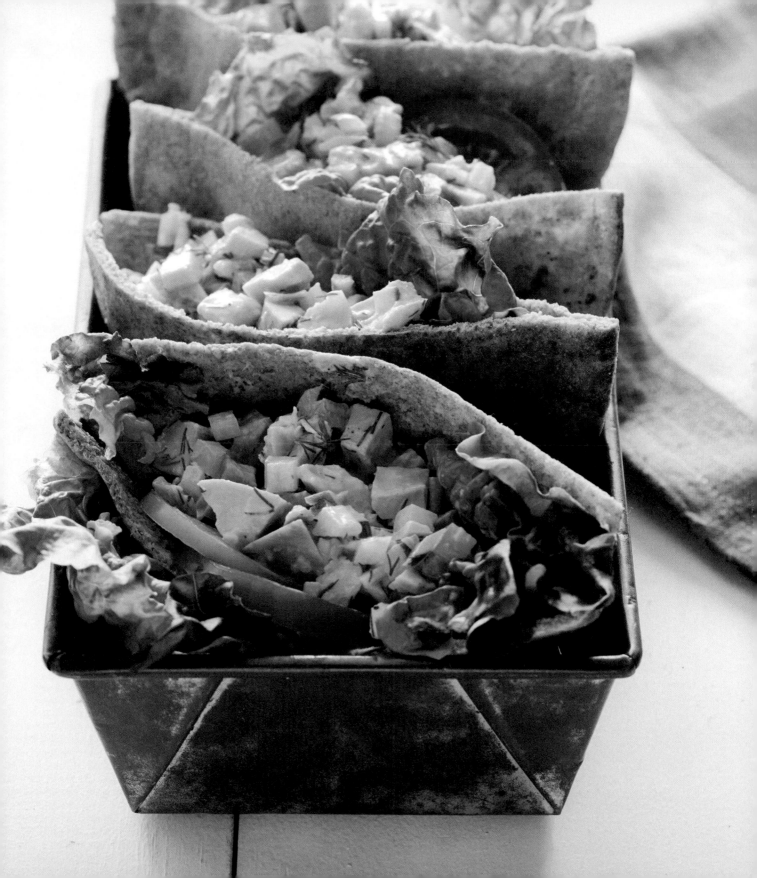

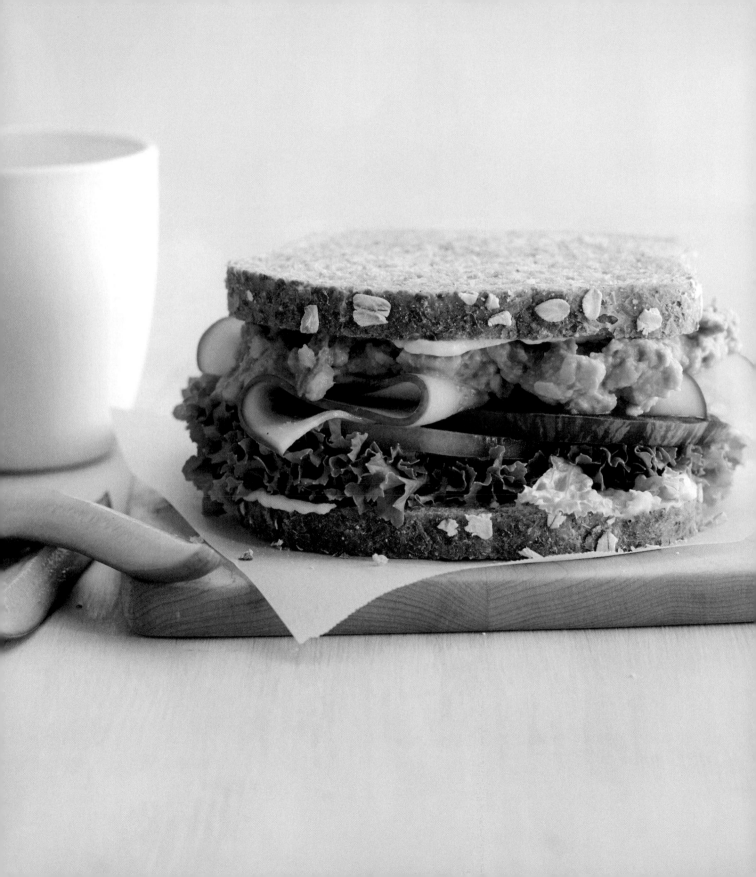

Avocado Sandwich

2 avocados, diced

2 teaspoons kosher or sea salt

Dash black pepper

Green leaf lettuce

1 Heirloom or beefsteak tomato, sliced

½ cucumber, thinly sliced lengthwise

Mustard greens (optional)

4 tablespoons organic or vegan mayonnaise

4 slices sprouted grain bread or gluten-free bread

This sandwich was inspired by the easy breezy days on the coast of California. Avocados are a wonderful and unusual fruit that contain good monounsaturated fats and powerful anti-inflammatory compounds.

DF **2 servings**

1. In a small bowl smash the avocado with the salt and pepper to make a chunky mixture that easily sticks together.

2. Spread mayonnaise evenly over each piece of bread. Layer one side with lettuce, mustard greens, tomato, and cucumber. Scoop half the smashed avocado evenly over the cucumber for each sandwich and top with second slice of bread. Repeat to make 2 sandwiches.

Food as Medicine

Avocados are rich in fiber, folate, vitamin E, vitamin K, and heart-healthy fat.

The Perfect Tuna Salad

2 (6-ounce) cans tuna, drained and flaked

⅓ cup organic or vegan mayonnaise

¼ cup diced celery

¼ cup diced sweet onion

1 hard-boiled egg, chopped

1 tablespoon pickle relish

1 teaspoon Dijon mustard

A tuna salad sandwich is a nutrient-rich one-dish meal, especially if it's topped with veggies. A mainstay of almost everyone's childhood, the tuna sandwich is loaded with protein and has more than 10% of your daily intake of 11 vitamins and minerals. Tuna is a good source of omega–3 fatty acids. Be sure to look for wild tuna that is low in mercury.

GF **DF** **4 servings**

Combine all ingredients in a medium bowl. Chill, if desired.

> **TIP** Keep this gluten free by creating a lettuce wrap or serving over mixed greens. Or serve on sprouted grain bread topped with two of your favorite sliced veggies.

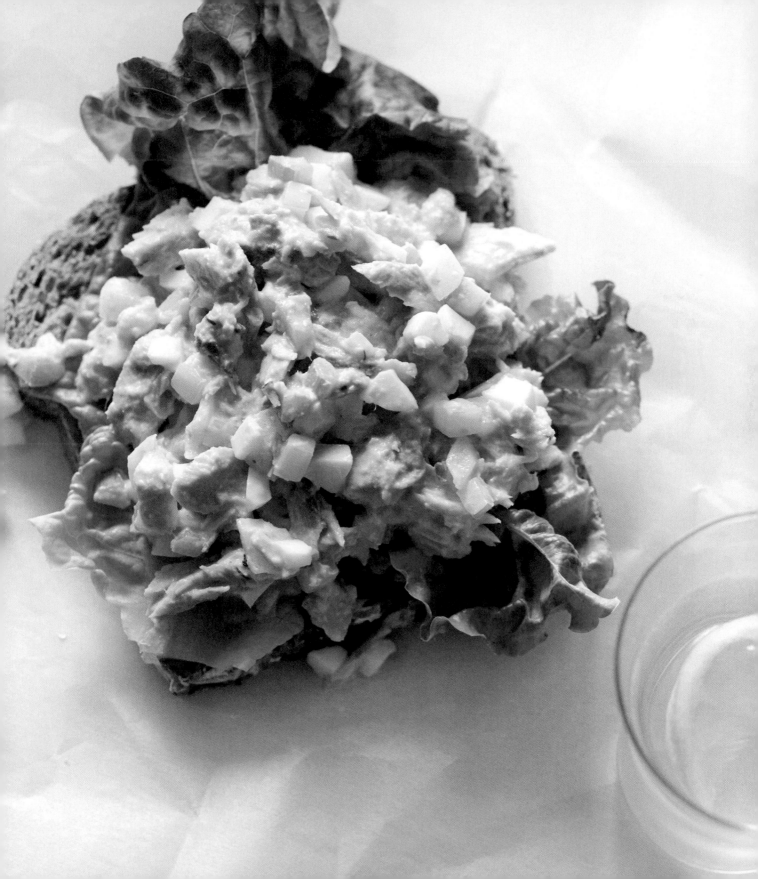

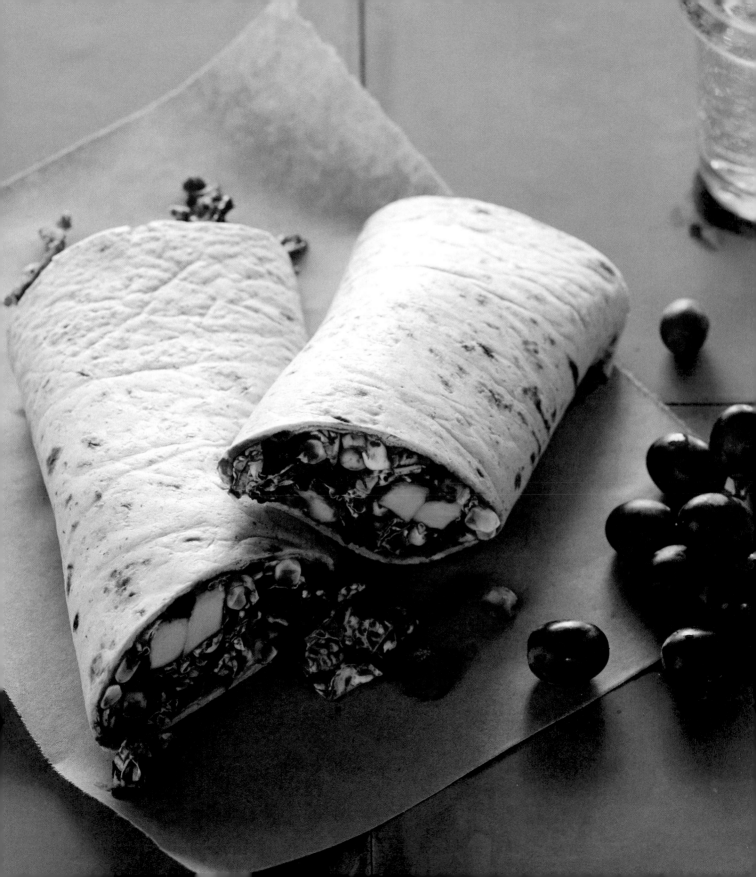

Chipotle Vegetable Wraps

2 brown rice, whole grain or 4 organic corn tortillas

Sauce

1 red bell pepper, diced

2 Roma tomatoes, diced

1 clove garlic, minced

1 chipotle pepper, dried (or 1 teaspoon chipotle powder)

2 tablespoons chili powder

1 teaspoon kosher or sea salt

⅓ cup water

3 tablespoons extra-virgin olive oil

Filling

⅔ cup shredded beets

⅔ cup shredded carrots

⅔ cup corn

1 avocado, cubed

2 cups finely chopped Napa cabbage or spinach

This simple wrap will become a go-to lunch favorite. Depending on your personal preference, use either gluten-free, whole grain, or organic corn tortillas. Simply prepare the vegetables based on how many people you are feeding, and you are ready to go! **DF** **V** **2 servings**

1. Combine bell pepper, tomatoes, garlic, pepper, chili powder, salt, and water in a blender. Blend until a thick vegetable puree forms. Add the olive oil, and mix well. Pour the sauce into an airtight container and store in the refrigerator (up to 4 days).

2. In a medium bowl, loosely toss the vegetables. Add ½ cup of the chipotle sauce, and toss until well coated. Divide the filling evenly between the wraps.

OPTIONAL If you prefer a warm wrap, place the entire wrap in an oven at 350° for 7 minutes to allow the wrap to crisp up.

Food as Medicine

Beets contain powerful cleansing agents for the liver and offer a wide range of vitamins and minerals. They also contain betaine, known to stimulate positive thoughts by supporting a balanced brain.

Chicken Lettuce Wraps

1 head iceberg lettuce, washed

Sauce

2 tablespoons water

1 tablespoon cornstarch

½ cup wheat-free tamari or soy sauce

2 tablespoons seasoned rice wine vinegar

2 tablespoons orange juice

½ teaspoon crushed red pepper

Filling

1 tablespoon coconut oil

1 teaspoon sesame oil

12 shitake or white button mushrooms, thinly sliced

1 large carrot, shredded

2 scallions, cut thinly on a diagonal

1 tablespoon finely chopped ginger

1 tablespoon finely chopped shallots

3 cloves garlic, minced

1 serrano pepper, seeded and minced

1 pound chicken breasts, cut into ½-inch pieces

1 small can of water chestnuts, drained, rinsed, and finely diced

¼ teaspoon black pepper

Lettuce wraps are becoming a new American classic. You can find them on many casual restaurant menus. Make your own Daniel Plan version at home for a fresh, nutritious lunch. **GF** **DF** **4 servings**

1. Combine water, cornstarch, tamari, vinegar, juice, and chile flakes in a jar or container. Seal lid tightly. Shake well. Set aside.

2. Place a large nonstick skillet over medium-high heat. When pan is hot, add coconut and sesame oils. Sauté mushrooms, carrots, scallion, ginger, shallots, garlic, and serrano pepper till tender, about 5 minutes.

3. Add chicken, and cook till chicken is almost done. Add the sauce, bring to a boil, then reduce heat to a simmer. Continue cooking 5–6 minutes. Remove pan from heat, and stir in water chestnuts and pepper.

4. Separate iceberg leaves to create lettuce cups. Spoon chicken mixture into lettuce cups, and serve immediately.

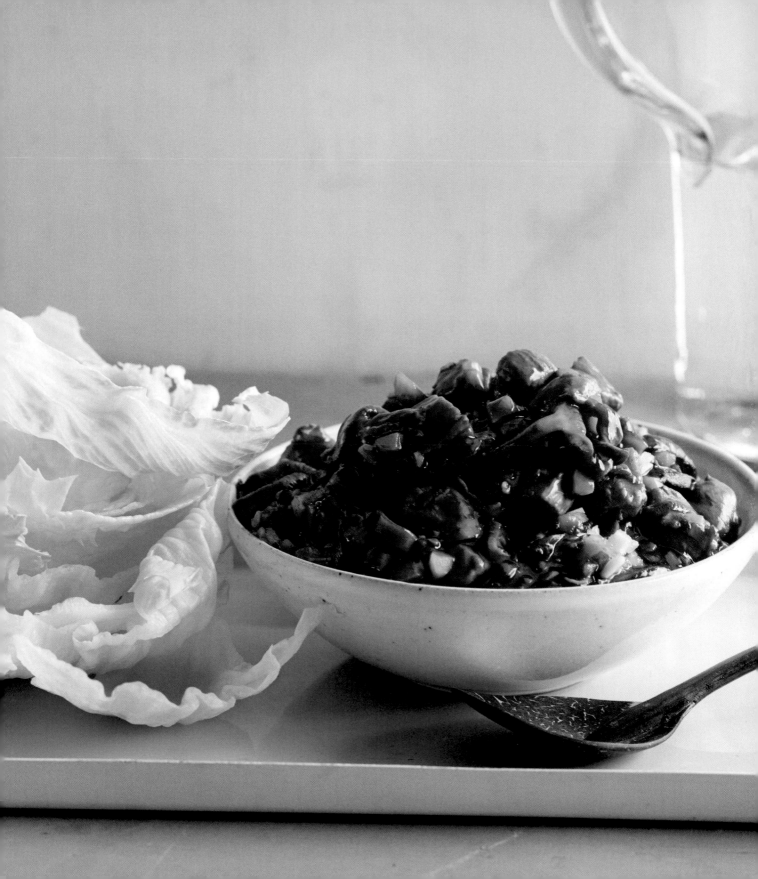

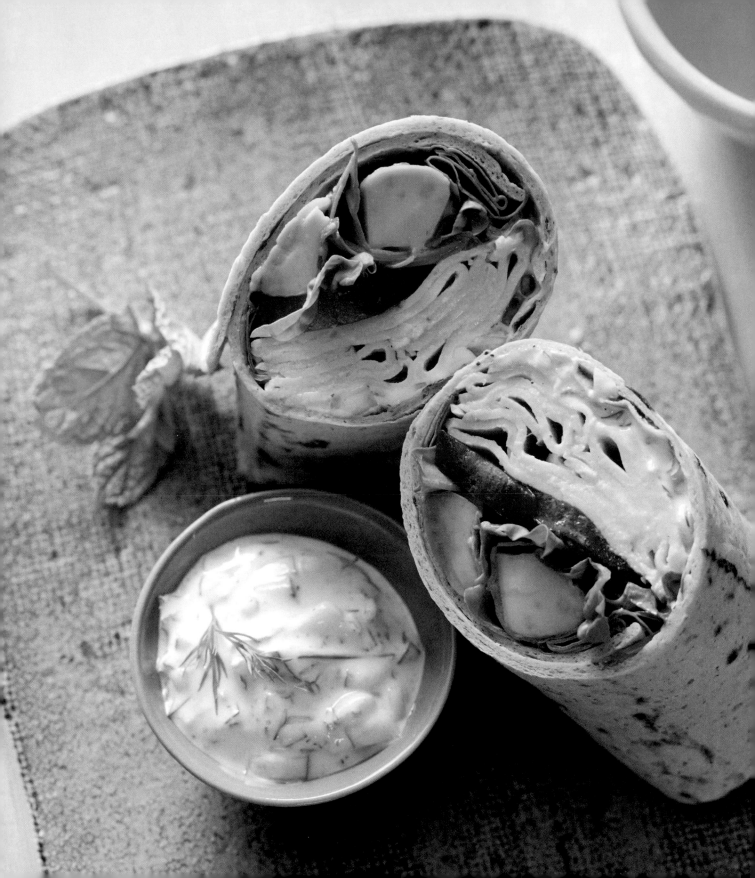

Turkey Veggie Wraps

4 large whole wheat or gluten-free wraps

½ cup Tzatziki Dip (page 173)

8 ounces thinly sliced deli-style turkey (nitrate-free)

1 large avocado, cut into eighths

2 tomatoes, sliced

4 small handfuls baby spinach leaves

Wraps make an easily transportable meal that contains a balanced Daniel Plan plate. For a grain-free version, wrap in large lettuce or Napa cabbage leaves.

DF 4 servings

1. Lay one wrap on a flat surface. Spread the wrap with a few tablespoons of the tzatziki.

2. Layer a few slices of turkey, avocado, tomatoes, and spinach. Roll and cut in half on the diagonal. Repeat to create four wraps.

3. Enjoy immediately, or wrap in plastic wrap and refrigerate for up to an hour.

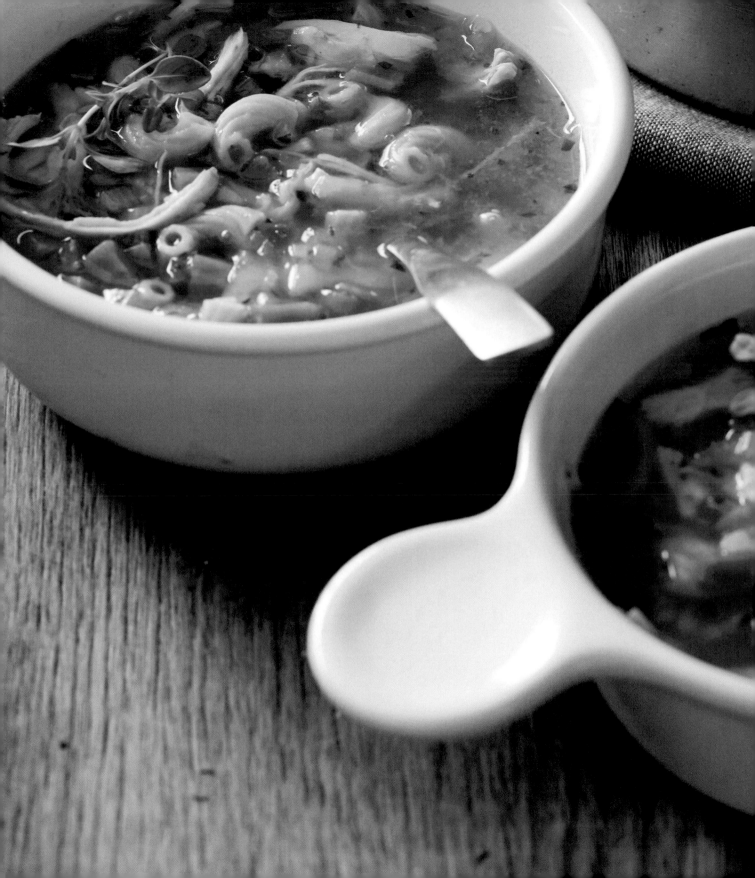

Soups, Stews, and Chilis

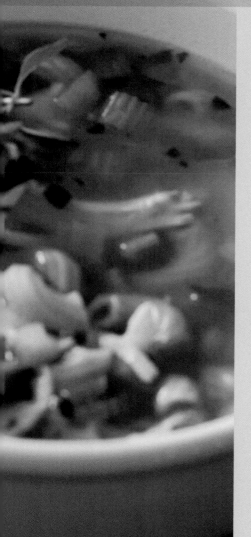

Chicken Noodle Vegetable Soup

2 tablespoons oil

3 ribs celery, finely chopped

2–3 carrots, finely chopped

1 medium onion, finely chopped

3 cloves garlic, minced

2 teaspoons minced fresh thyme (or ¾ teaspoon dried thyme)

1 bay leaf

Kosher or sea salt and black pepper

1 large bone-in chicken breast (or 2–3 cups cooked chicken)

2 quarts (64 ounces) low-sodium chicken broth

1 cup whole wheat or brown rice elbow pasta

1 tablespoon fresh parsley, chopped

Classic and comforting, nothing is better than homemade chicken soup. It can be made in about an hour, even less if you use leftover shredded roasted chicken and pre-cooked pasta. To make this gluten-free, use brown rice pasta.

DF **4–6 servings**

1. Add oil to a large pot over medium heat. Turn the heat down to medium-low and add the celery, carrots, and onion. Cook until the vegetables are soft and translucent, 12–15 minutes. Stir in the garlic, and cook another 30–60 seconds. Add thyme, bay leaf, salt, and pepper.

2. Remove skin and fat from chicken breast. Cut chicken breast crosswise through the bone into two pieces. Add the broth and the chicken breast to the pot. Bring to a boil, reduce to a simmer, and cook until chicken is cooked through, about 18 minutes.

3. Remove chicken from the pot. Add the pasta to the hot water, and simmer until pasta is tender (check package instructions). When chicken is cool enough to handle, shred the meat, and add back to the pot to warm.

4. Remove the bay leaf. Add parsley. Ladle into warm bowls to serve.

Spicy Black Bean Soup with Lime and Cilantro

1 tablespoon extra-virgin olive oil

1 tablespoon minced garlic

1 jalapeno pepper, seeded, minced

1 large red onion, diced

1 large tomato, seeded and diced

1 tablespoon chili powder

1 tablespoon cumin

1 bay leaf

½ teaspoon chipotle powder

2 teaspoons fresh oregano

2 (15-ounce) cans black beans, drained and rinsed

2 (14-ounce) cans vegetable broth

1 lime cut into wedges

1 cup finely chopped fresh cilantro

Black bean soup is a great alternative to meat-based chilis. Beans are powerhouse foods that pack protein, fiber, and vitamins — and they are budget-friendly. **GF** **DF** **V** **4 – 6 servings**

1. Heat olive oil in a large stockpot over medium-high heat. Add garlic, jalapeno, and onion. Sauté till tender, about 5 minutes. Add tomato, and continue cooking another 5 minutes or until the onion is translucent.

2. Add chili powder, cumin, bay leaf, chipotle powder, oregano, black beans, and vegetable broth. Stir. Bring to a boil, then reduce heat to medium-low, and let soup simmer for at least 10 minutes.

3. Remove bay leaf. Either serve this soup as is, or use an immersion blender or traditional blender (blending in small batches) to puree the soup. Serve warm, and garnish with a squeeze of fresh lime and some fresh chopped cilantro.

TIP   Dried beans are less expensive than canned but require prep time. You must soak dried beans before cooking. Either cover with water and soak overnight or boil beans with a few cups of water for 2 minutes, then remove from heat, cover, and let stand for 2 hours.

Asparagus Crème Soup

2 cups diced asparagus

½ cup diced white or brown onion

2 tablespoons extra-virgin olive oil

2 cups dried split peas

6 cups water

2 cloves garlic

Kosher or sea salt

Black pepper

This is a high-protein soup made creamy by the use of split peas. It's a surefire comfort food and makes a nice accompaniment to any number of dishes from salad to grilled salmon. **GF** **DF** **V**   **4 servings**

1. In a medium to large stock pot over medium heat, lightly toss the asparagus, onions, and olive oil for 4 minutes.

2. Add in remaining ingredients. Bring the mixture to boiling, then cover and let simmer on medium heat for 25 minutes, stirring every 5–7 minutes to prevent the mixture from sticking to the bottom of the pot. Remove from the heat.

3. Using an immersion blender or in small batches in a regular blender, blend the mixture until rich and creamy. Leftovers will keep for 3 days in the refrigerator. Reheat it over medium heat and add ⅓ cup water.

Food as Medicine
Peas are a great source of minerals and protein. They provide a healthy supply of iron and folate and are anti-inflammatory. Pass the peas, please!

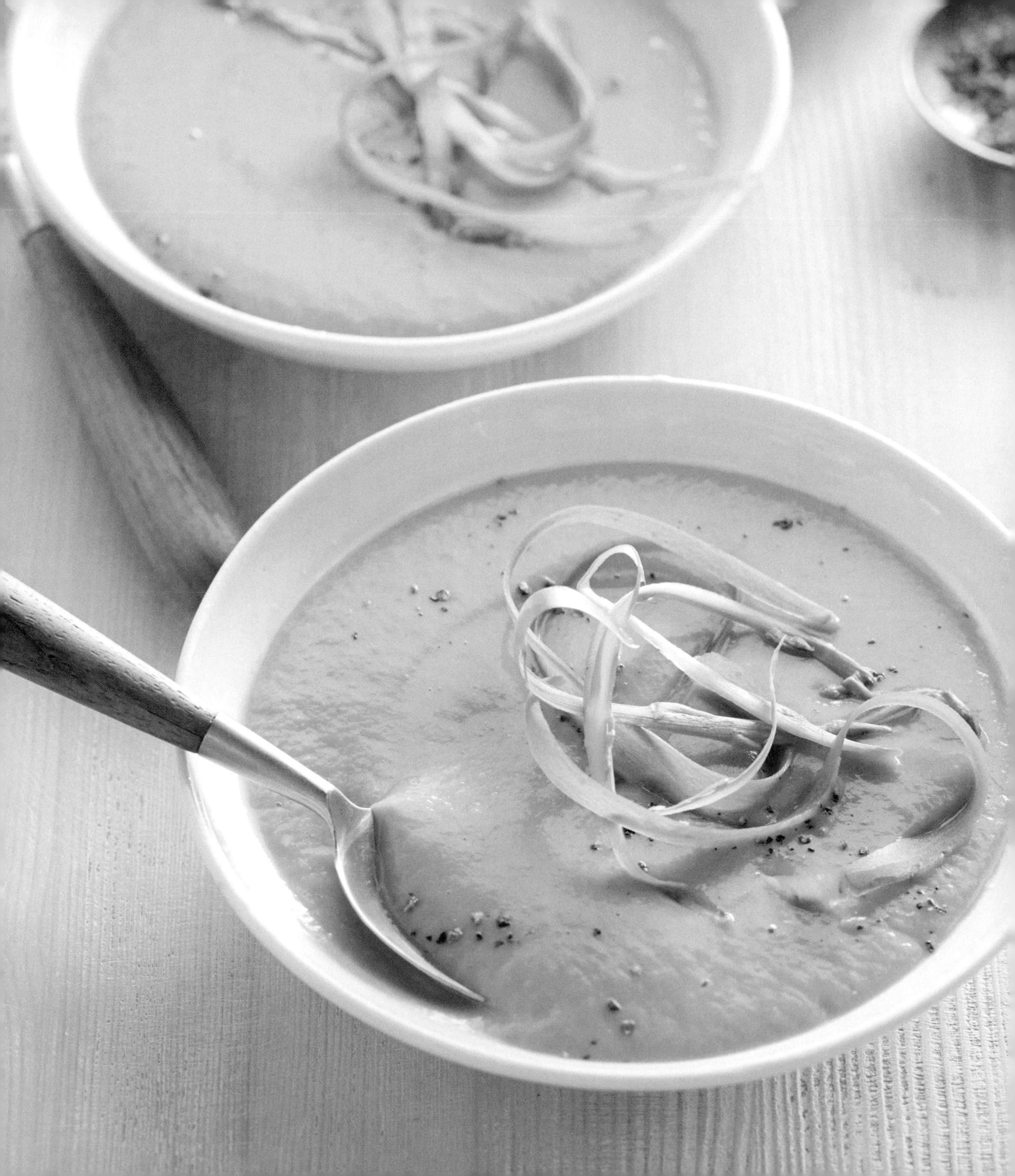

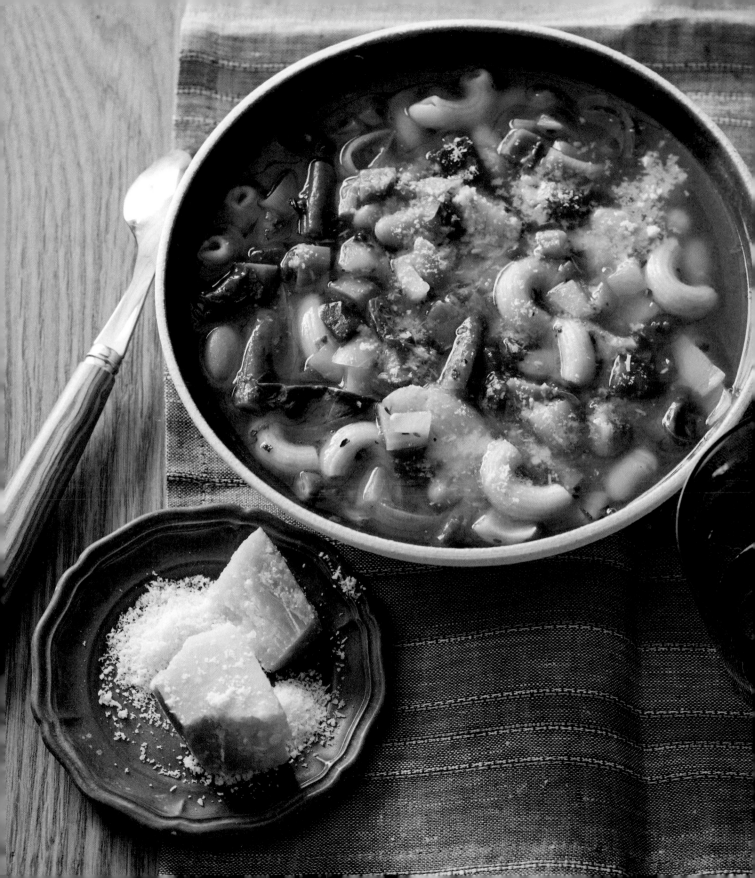

Vegetable Minestrone

1 large leek

1 medium fennel bulb

3 carrots, scrubbed

1 red or yellow bell pepper

2 tablespoons extra-virgin olive oil

3–4 cloves garlic, minced

½ teaspoon kosher or sea salt

¼ teaspoon black pepper

1 tablespoon mixed dried Italian herbs (oregano, rosemary, thyme, basil)

1 (15-ounce) can petite-diced tomatoes, drained

8 cups (2 quarts) low-sodium chicken or vegetable broth

½ cup whole wheat or brown rice elbow pasta

1 cup fresh green beans, chopped

1 (15-ounce) can Cannellini beans, rinsed and drained

1 large handful fresh baby spinach

Minestrone means "big soup" in Italian, and this soup is big on fresh vegetables and flavors. You'll get good knife practice chopping the vegetables, but don't let that deter you. This soup is a meal in a bowl. DF V **6–8 servings**

1. Cut the dark green top and the root off the leek. Slice the remaining leek in half lengthwise, and rinse away any sand or grit under cold running water. Chop leek into thin half moons.

2. Cut off the top stems and fronds of the fennel bulb. Trim a thin slice off the bottom. Slice the bulb in half from top to bottom. Cut out the pyramid-shaped core. Chop the halves into long, thin pieces, then chop crosswise.

3. Scrub and chop carrots (peeling removes vitamins and minerals that are in the skin) and bell pepper into small pieces, about ½-inch in size.

4. In a large pot over medium heat, add olive oil. When oil is hot, add the leek, fennel, carrot, and bell pepper. Stir. Add the dried herbs. Reduce to low, and cover with a lid. Cook until vegetables are soft, stirring occasionally, about 12–15 minutes.

5. Remove the lid and stir in the garlic. Cook 30 seconds. Add salt and pepper. (Add more later if needed.)

6. Add tomatoes and broth to the pot. Turn up heat, and bring almost to a boil, then reduce to a simmer. Add the pasta and green beans. Cook partially covered with the lid until the pasta is tender. Add the beans and spinach. Heat for 5 minutes. (Sprinkle with Parmesan.)

CANNELLINI BEANS are white kidney beans. You can substitute red kidney, great northern, or Navy beans.

Lentil-Quinoa Soup

1 cup dried quinoa

1½ cups dried lentils

6 cups vegetable stock

1 Roma tomato, diced

1 onion, diced

1 cup diced celery

2 cups diced carrots

2 cloves garlic, minced

1 tablespoon kosher
or sea salt

Black pepper

⅓ cup fresh parsley
(optional)

Lentils and quinoa are both a good source of plant protein. This is a good recipe for integrating vegetable scraps from other food preparations. The more the merrier when it comes to adding vegetables to this soup!

GF DF V   **4 servings**

1. Cook the quinoa according to the package instructions. Set aside.

2. Combine lentils, stock, tomato, onion, celery, carrots, garlic, salt, and pepper in a large stockpot or a crock-pot. If using a stockpot, bring the mixture to a boil, then reduce heat, and let simmer covered for approximately 30 minutes. Stir the soup every 15 minutes or so to prevent lentils from sticking.

3. Add the quinoa. Stir the mixture well, cover the pot, and cook on low heat for another 15 minutes.

4. If using a crock-pot, place ingredients in the pot, and place on low heat for 4–6 hours, depending on your piece of equipment. When ready to enjoy, place the quinoa into the pot, stir well, and let sit for 15 minutes before serving.

5. Garnish with fresh parsley and pepper. This soup will keep for 3 days in the refrigerator.

Food as Medicine

Lentils are a superfood that boosts metabolism and provides satiating fiber and protein. Quinoa contains all 9 essential amino acids, almost twice as much fiber as other grains, plus iron, lysine, magnesium, riboflavin, and manganese.

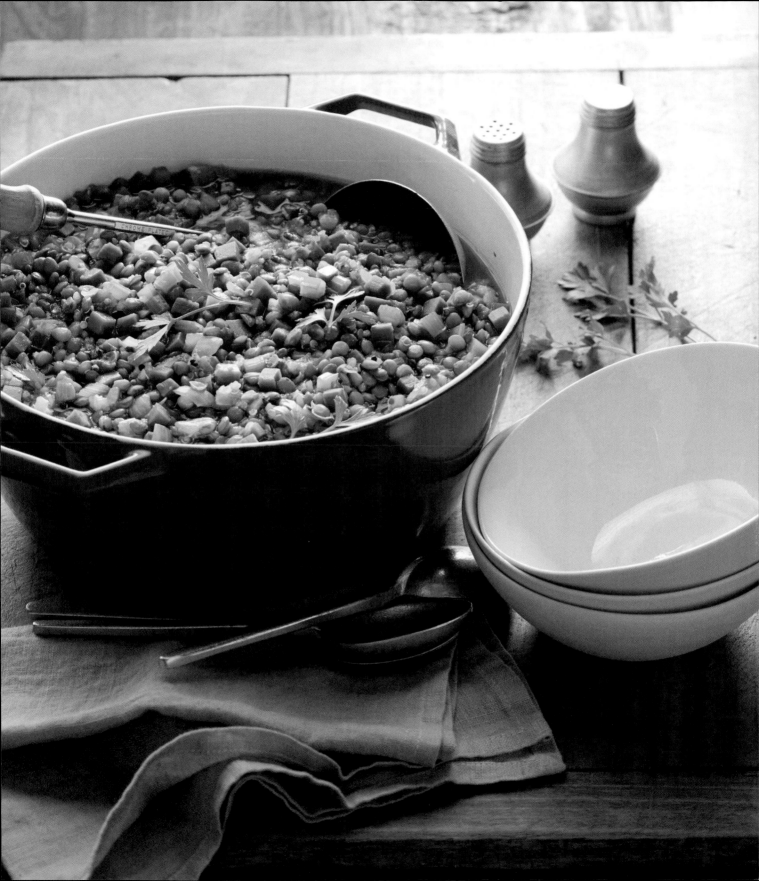

Manhattan Beach Seafood Chowder

2 tablespoons grape
seed oil

1 cup diced sweet onion

1 cup diced leeks

1 cup diced celery

½ cup diced carrot

½ cup diced green bell
pepper

3 garlic cloves, minced

1 (6-ounce) can tomato
paste

1 cup water

2 cups diced red potatoes

2 cups tomatoes

1 (28-ounce) can diced
tomatoes

2 cups water

1 tablespoon dried thyme

1 teaspoon kosher
or sea salt

½ teaspoon black pepper

2 cups clam juice

1 bay leaf

½ pound shrimp, peeled
and deveined

½ pound halibut, skinned,
cut into 1-inch squares

½ pound salmon, skinned,
cut into 1-inch squares

½ pound cod, skinned, cut
into 1-inch squares (or any
fish you like)

According to the American Heart Association, we should eat 2 servings of fish per week to prevent coronary heart disease. Fish and shellfish are excellent sources of lean protein, low in saturated fat, and high in essential omega-3 fatty acids. **GF DF** **4–6 servings**

1. In a large soup or stock pot over medium-high heat, heat oil. Sauté onion, leek, celery, carrot, bell pepper, and garlic till soft, about 12–15 minutes or until lightly browned.

2. Stir in tomato paste; cook 1 minute. Add water, stir, and bring to a boil. Simmer 5 minutes.

3. Add potatoes, all tomatoes, water, thyme, salt, pepper, clam juice, and bay leaf. Bring to a boil. Reduce heat; simmer 30 minutes.

4. Add fish. Cover and simmer 10 minutes or until fish flakes easily when tested with a fork. Discard bay leaf.

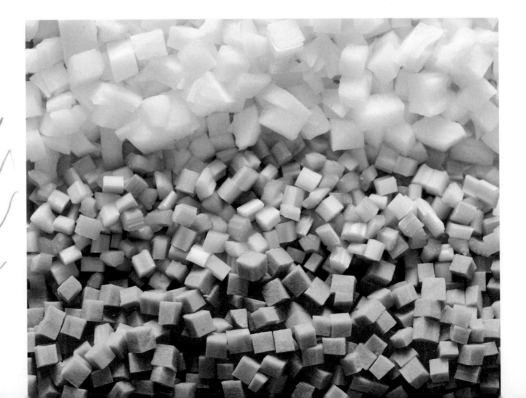

Red Lentil Stew

2 tablespoons extra-virgin olive oil

½ onion, diced

2 tablespoons minced garlic

2 teaspoons black or yellow mustard seeds

1 teaspoon cumin

1 teaspoon turmeric

½ teaspoon coriander

1 small carrot, diced

2 cups cauliflower, cut into small florets

1¼ cups red (or brown) lentils, rinsed

6 cups water

1 cup diced tomato

2 cups broccoli, cut into small florets

½ teaspoon kosher or sea salt

1 tablespoon lemon juice

Chopped fresh parsley or cilantro (optional)

Dr. Hyman Favorite

Lentil stew has been around for thousands of years. Jacob served it to his brother Esau and started a family feud. Fortunately, this version will gather people around your table and provide a healthy and hearty meal that everyone will enjoy. The original version of this stew appeared in *The Blood Sugar Solution* by Mark Hyman, M.D.

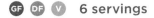 **6 servings**

1. Heat olive oil in a large soup pot over medium heat. Sauté onions and garlic until tender. Add mustard seeds, and stir until they begin to pop. Add other spices, and sauté 1 minute. Add carrot and cauliflower, and stir to coat.

2. Add lentils and water. Bring to a boil. Reduce heat to low, and simmer until lentils are soft, about 25 minutes. Add tomato, broccoli, and salt. Simmer 5 more minutes.

3. Just before serving, stir in lemon juice and sprinkle with parsley or cilantro.

Food as Medicine

Curcumin is found in the yellow spice called turmeric and is used in curries and mustards.
It is nature's ibuprofen and a powerful anti-inflammatory.

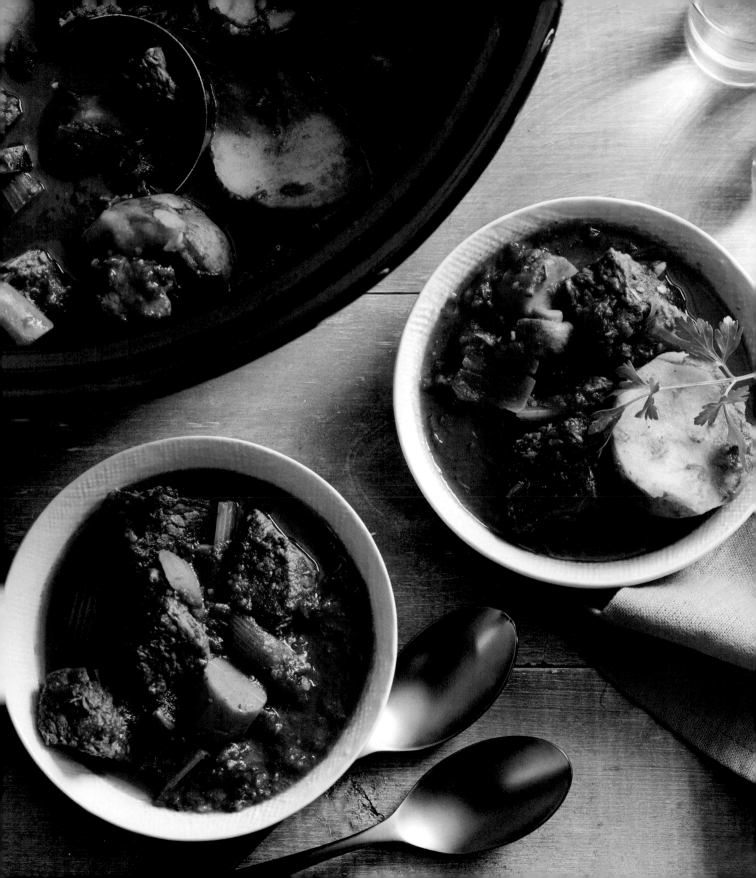

Crock-Pot Beef Stew

Olive or grape seed oil

1½ pounds lean beef top round, cut into 1½-inch cubes

½ teaspoon black pepper

1 teaspoon fresh thyme

1 teaspoon minced fresh parsley

1 medium red onion, diced

2 garlic cloves, minced

1 large (28-ounce) can crushed tomatoes

2 stalks celery, cut into 1-inch pieces

2 medium carrots, cut into 1-inch pieces

½ pound mushrooms, cut in half

1 tablespoon wheat-free tamari or soy sauce

2 cups low-sodium beef broth

6 small redskin potatoes, cut in quarters

A few good reasons to use your crock-pot? It makes the house smell good, it's easy to clean up, and it makes a lot of food. A crock-pot is an economical way to make large one-dish meals. Here's one perfect for Sunday supper. **GF** **DF** **4 – 6 servings**

1. Coat a soup or stock pot with oil, and place over medium heat.

2. Season beef with black pepper. Brown beef for 4–5 minutes.

3. Place the thyme, parsley, onion, garlic, crushed tomatoes, diced celery, carrots, mushrooms, tamari sauce, and beef broth in the crock-pot. Add the seasoned beef. Turn heat on low. Cover and simmer until slightly tender about 6–7 hours.

4. Add potatoes to crock-pot. Add water if stew is looking dry. Simmer about 3–4 more hours on low.

TIP You can also bake the stew in the oven at 325° for 6–7 hours or on the stove top over medium heat, covered for 5–6 hours.

Warm-You-Up Chicken Stew

2 tablespoons extra-virgin olive oil

3 skinless bone-in chicken breasts

1 medium yellow onion, chopped

2 stalks celery, cut into 1-inch pieces

1 quart low-sodium vegetable stock or chicken stock

2 medium carrots, peeled and cut into ½-inch pieces

2 medium turnips, peeled and cut into ½-inch pieces

3 medium Yukon gold potatoes, peeled and quartered

½ teaspoon fresh thyme

½ teaspoon chopped fresh basil

½ teaspoon fresh tarragon

Kosher or sea salt and black pepper

Nothing is more inviting than a warm bowl of stew on a chilly night. In this dish, a variety of herbs boosts the flavor and aroma as well as the nutritional value in every spoonful. **GF** **DF**   **6 servings**

1. Heat olive oil in a large pot over medium high heat.

2. Sprinkle chicken with salt and pepper on both sides. Place chicken pieces, meat side down, in oil and cook for 2–3 minutes on each side.

3. Add the onions, celery, and stock. Bring to a simmer, lower heat, cover, and simmer gently for about 45 minutes, until chicken is done.

4. Add the rest of the vegetables and the herbs. Bring to a boil. Reduce heat to a gentle simmer for about 10 minutes or until the vegetables are almost fork tender.

5. Remove chicken pieces, cool slightly, and pull meat from the bones. Break meat into large pieces. Return meat to pot, and cook uncovered until vegetables are very tender, about 15 minutes. Season with salt and pepper.

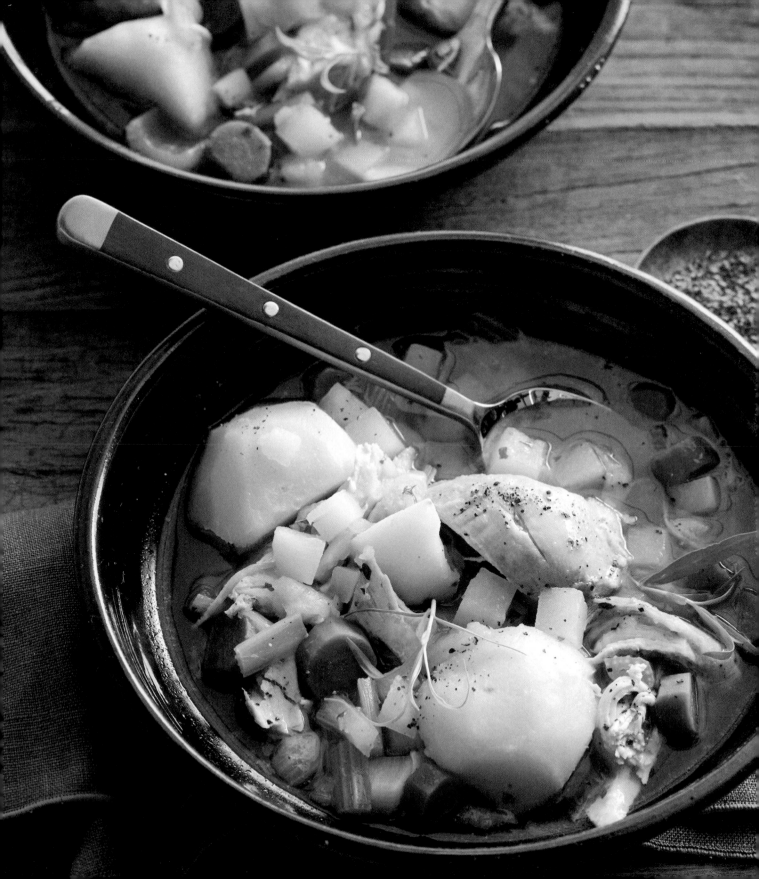

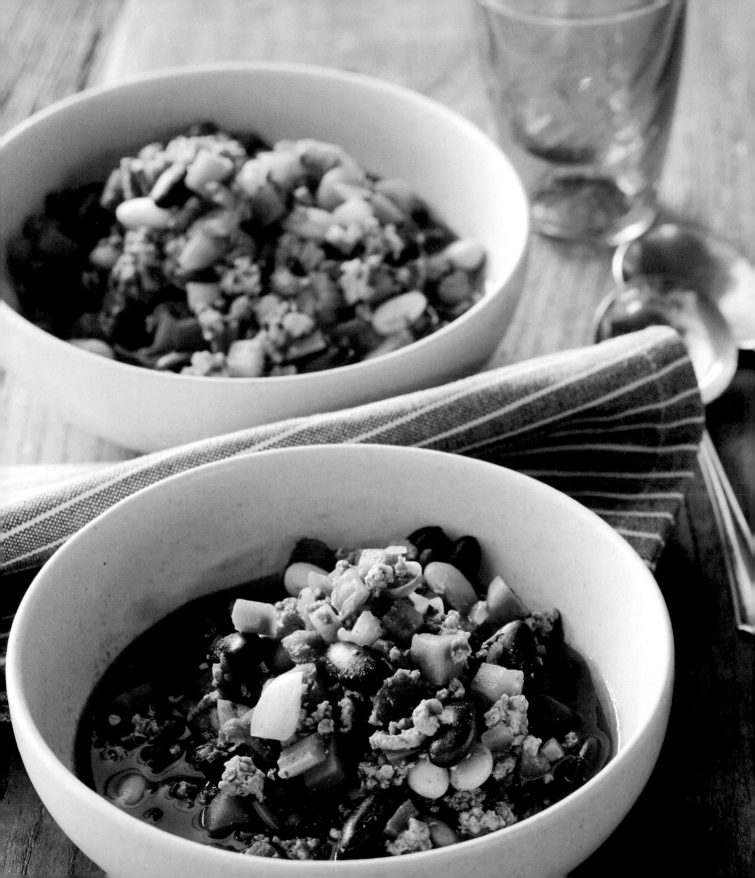

Turkey-Bean Chili

1 tablespoon extra-virgin olive oil

1 cup finely chopped celery

1 cup finely chopped carrots

½ green bell pepper, finely chopped

1 cup finely chopped red onion

2 tablespoons tomato paste

3 large garlic cloves, minced

1 pound ground turkey

1 tablespoon mild chili powder

1 teaspoon cumin

2 teaspoons dried oregano

½ teaspoon Kosher or sea salt

¼ teaspoon black pepper

1 (15-ounce) can diced tomatoes (try fire-roasted)

1 (15-ounce) can red kidney beans, rinsed and drained

1 (15-ounce) can Cannellini or white Navy beans, rinsed and drained

1 cup low-sodium chicken or vegetable broth

Don't let the list of ingredients deter you from making this tasty chili. It comes together in about 30 minutes. One way to improve efficiency is to get all your ingredients out and ready for cooking. This practice is called *mise en place*, a French cooking term for everything in its place.

GF DF **4–6 servings**

1. In a large pot, heat the olive oil over medium heat. Add celery, carrot, bell pepper, and onion. Cook until soft, stirring occasionally. If vegetables start to brown, turn the heat down a bit.

2. Add tomato paste, and cook 2 minutes stirring continuously. Add garlic, and cook 1 minute.

3. Add turkey to the pot. Break up turkey with the back of a wooden spoon or spatula while it cooks. Cook until turkey is no longer pink. Add chili powder, cumin, oregano, salt, and pepper. Cook 2 minutes, allowing spices to release their flavors. Stir once or twice.

4. Add the tomatoes, beans, and broth. Cover and heat until chili is hot and bubbly.

CHILI POWDER is usually a blend of Ancho chile pepper, cumin, garlic, and Mexican oregano. Some blends add red pepper for heat or ground chipotle for heat and a smoky flavor.

Vegan Chili on Smashed Yams

Chili

1 (15-ounce) can black beans

1 (15-ounce) can pinto beans

1 (15-ounce) can kidney beans

⅓ cup chili powder

2 tomatoes, diced

1 onion, finely chopped

1 chipotle pepper (optional)

4 tablespoons extra-virgin olive oil

1 tablespoon kosher or sea salt

6 cups water

Potatoes

6 cups diced yams or Yukon gold potatoes

2 quarts water

4 tablespoons organic or vegan mayonnaise

1 teaspoon chili powder

2 tablespoons extra-virgin olive oil

1 teaspoon kosher or sea salt

6 scallions, diced (optional)

2 tomatoes, diced (optional)

3–4 tablespoons shredded cheese (omit for V) or cheese alternative

This dish is fulfilling and perfect for any time of the year. The chili is high in protein; serve it as a side with any number of dishes or enjoy it alone. This is a perfect dish to prepare at the beginning of the week so you have leftovers for other meals. **GF** **DF** **V** **6 servings**

1. Put all ingredients for the chili into a crock-pot. Cook on medium or high for 4 hours. Or put all ingredients into a stockpot on the stove, and bring to a boil. Let boil for 3–4 minutes. Then reduce heat to a simmer and cover. Simmer for 35 minutes.

2. When the chili is almost done, fill a medium pan with 2 quarts water. Add a dash of salt. Bring water to a boil. Add the yams to the boiling water. Reduce heat to a simmer and cook for 20 minutes, or until potatoes are soft all the way through.

3. Strain the potatoes in a colander, and rinse lightly. Transfer the potatoes to a mixing bowl, and add the mayonnaise, chili powder, oil, and salt. Lightly smash the potatoes using a fork or spatula, loosely combining all ingredients in the bowl.

4. Scoop out 1 cup of potatoes, and serve with 1 cup of chili. Top with scallions, diced tomatoes, and 1 tablespoon shredded cheese or cheese alternative.

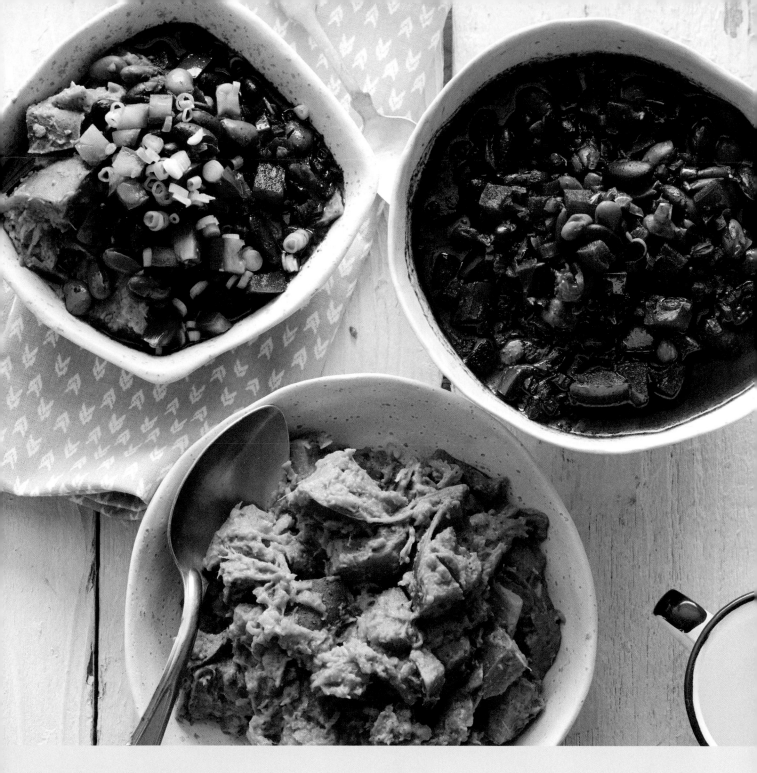

Food as Medicine

Yams are a great source of B6 vitamins and potassium. Yams are sometimes confused with sweet potatoes. Yams grow in a variety of colors and over 200 different varieties. They are usually long and skinny.

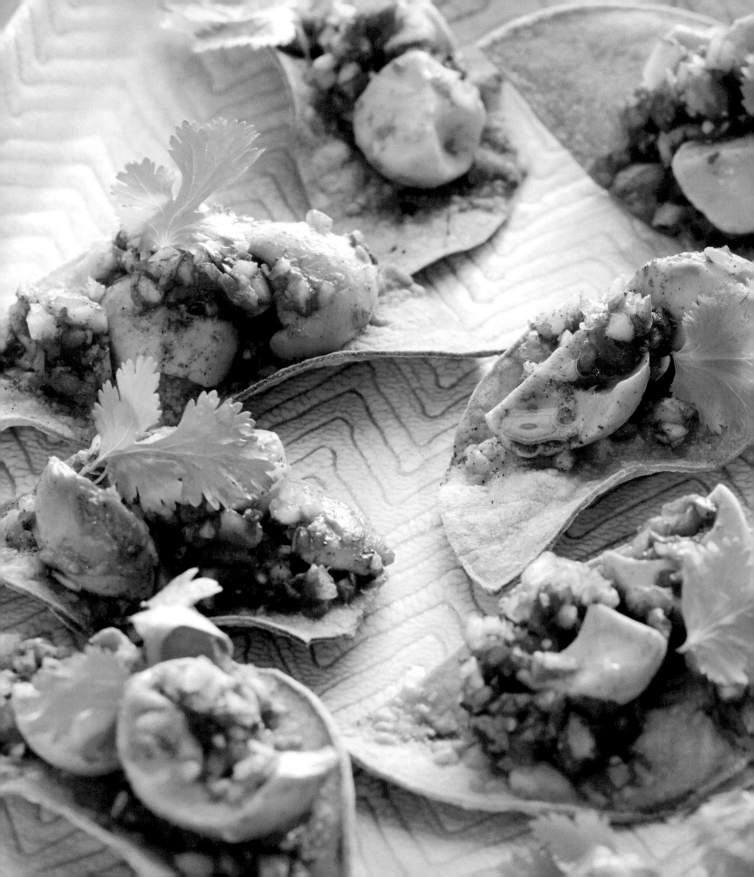

Snacks and Appetizers

Chips and Guacamole with Fresh Salsa

Corn chips

1 package organic corn tortillas

1 lime wedge

1 tablespoon chili-garlic salt or sea salt

Guacamole

2 avocados, halved

1 teaspoon kosher or sea salt

1 lemon or lime

Black pepper

¼ cup chopped cilantro (optional)

Cayenne or jalapeno pepper (optional)

Salsa

4 tomatoes, diced

2 green onions

⅓ cup fresh cilantro

½ cup lemon juice

1 teaspoon kosher or sea salt

1 serrano pepper (optional)

A classic favorite as a snack or a starter, this dish has a few twists. We have worked around the classic chip to create an easy baked version that is just as crunchy and flavorful. For the salsa, we have given you a basic recipe to work from — be creative with it to suit your tastes.

GF **DF** **V**   **4 servings**

1. Preheat the oven to 350°.

2. Cut corn tortillas in quarters or eighths. In a medium bowl, toss the tortillas with the lime juice. Then sprinkle the chili-garlic salt or sea salt over the bowl, and toss again. If needed, use your fingers to disperse the salt loosely over the tortilla pieces.

3. Line up the tortilla pieces on a baking sheet so they do not overlap. Place in the oven for 7 minutes. Remove the baking sheet and use tongs to flip over each chip. Place back in the oven for 7–10 minutes until they are crispy.

4. Remove from the oven and let cool. These chips will store in an airtight container for up to 2 weeks.

5. In a food processor, add all salsa ingredients and pulse to desired consistency. Remove the salsa from the food processor and refrigerate until ready for use. This salsa will keep for 3 days in the refrigerator.

6. In a small bowl, place the sea salt and avocado. Using the back side of a fork, smash the avocado over and over until a chunky avocado spread has formed. Now squeeze the lemon or lime over the avocado and sprinkle with salt and pepper. Stir into the mixture. If you enjoy a little heat, add cayenne or jalapeno pepper, tasting as you go until it has reached the desired flavor. Garnish with fresh cilantro.

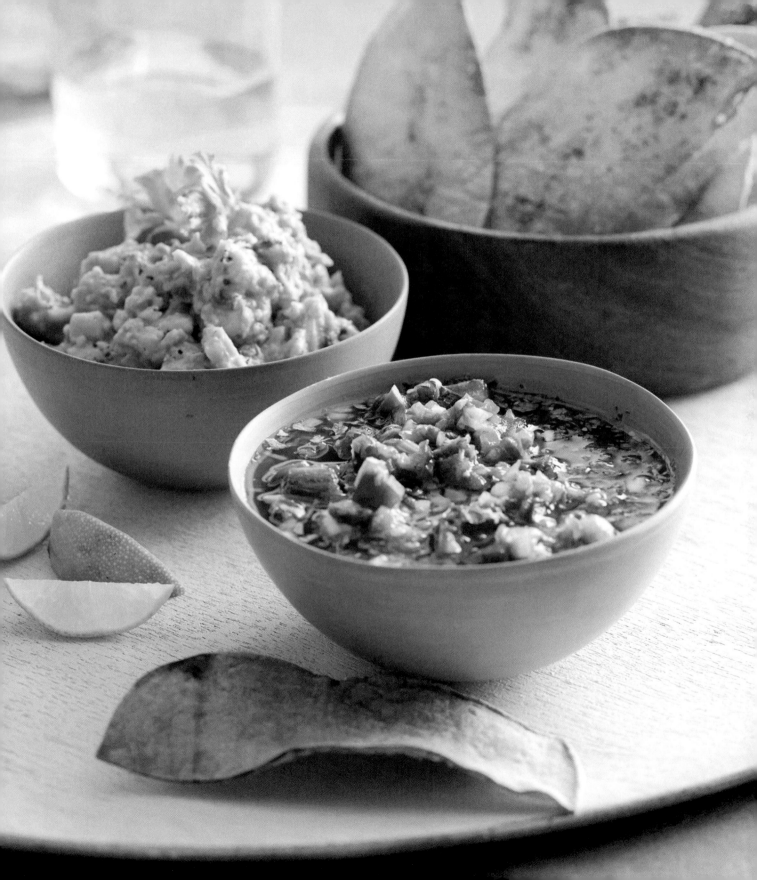

Kale Chips

2 heads kale

½ cup tahini paste

2 tablespoons nutritional yeast

½ cup lemon juice

1 tablespoon kosher or sea salt

1 teaspoon cayenne pepper (optional)

Don't let the hardiness of kale or the appearance of kale chips scare you away. Turning this powerhouse veggie into a quick, crispy, and nutritious snack will make you a fan. This recipe works well with curly kale or lacinato kale with the stems removed. Take it on faith—once you try this guilt-free snack, you may never go back to potato chips.

GF **DF** **V**   **4 servings**

1. Preheat the oven to 350°.

2. Rinse kale well and dry. Remove the stems by pulling the leaves back from the stem, "stripping" away the leaves. Cut the leaves down to roughly 4-inch segments.

3. In a small mixing bowl, whisk together the tahini, yeast, lemon juice, salt, and cayenne. Gently pour this mixture over the kale, and toss until all the kale is well coated.

4. Place the leaves on a baking sheet. Bake for about 20 minutes. Check the kale often as each head of kale has different water content. Sometimes kale will cook up quickly if it is already dry. The chips should be crispy. Store them in an airtight jar or container.

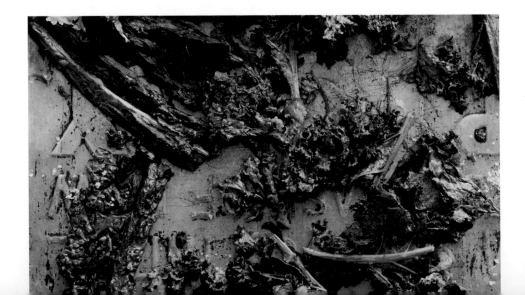

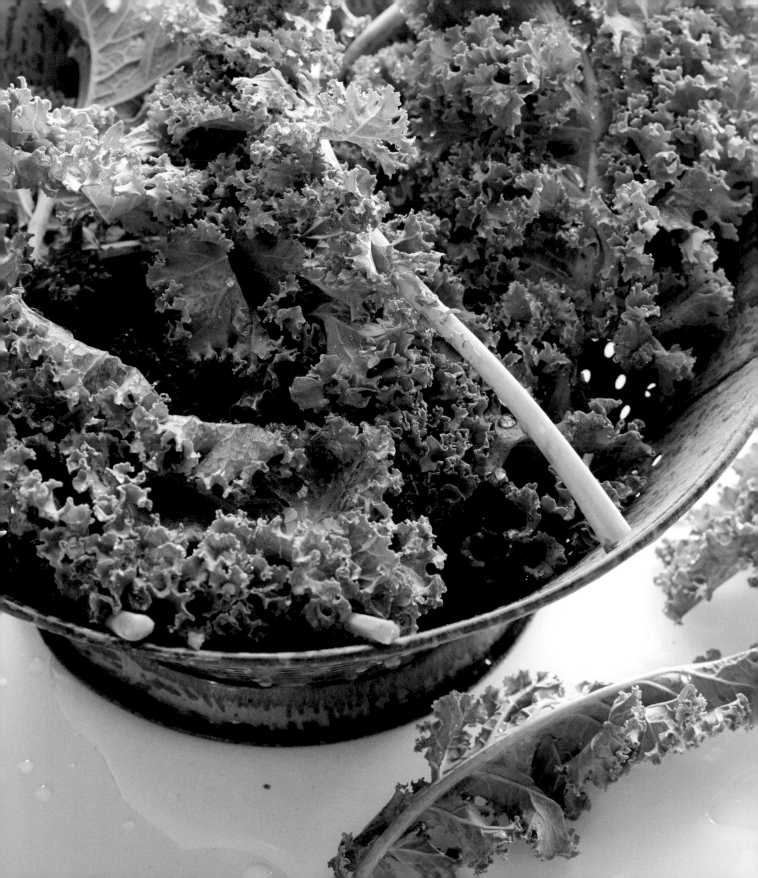

Mediterranean Hummus

1 (15-ounce) can garbanzo beans, rinsed and drained

½ cup oil-packed sun-dried tomatoes

10–12 pitted Kalamata olives

2 tablespoons extra-virgin olive oil (or oil from the tomato jar)

1 tablespoon chopped fresh basil

1 tablespoon chopped fresh oregano

Juice of 1 lemon

1 large garlic clove, minced

Kosher or sea salt

Black pepper

With ingredients typical of the Mediterranean — Greek olives, Italian herbs, sun-dried tomatoes, and olive oil — this hummus is anything but standard. Serve with raw vegetables, crackers, or pita wedges. **GF DF V** **6–8 servings**

1. Place the beans, tomatoes, olives, oil, herbs, juice, and garlic in the bowl of a food processor. Process until smooth.

2. Taste, then season with salt, pepper, and a few more herbs if you like.

TIP This is a thick hummus. If you want it creamier, add a little more oil or warm water to achieve your preferred consistency.

Food as Medicine
Nutritional yeast is a supplement that can be used to create a "cheese-like" flavor in sauces and spreads. Most varieties contain 400% of the nutritional requirement of vitamin B-12.

Top to bottom: Mediterranean Hummus,
Roasted Red Hummus (page 172),
Mexican-Style Hummus (page 172)

Mexican-Style Hummus

1 (15-ounce) can garbanzo
beans, rinsed and drained

1 (4-ounce) can roasted mild
green chiles, drained

1 tablespoon tahini (sesame
seed paste)

2 tablespoons extra-virgin
olive oil

2 tablespoons chopped fresh
cilantro

Juice of 1–2 limes

2 large garlic cloves, minced

2 teaspoons cumin

1 teaspoon coriander

½ teaspoon kosher or sea salt

¼ teaspoon black pepper

This creamy, bean-based dip has South-of-the-Border flavors. Use your food processor to whip it together in just minutes. Serve with baked tortilla chips or jicama and bell pepper strips.

GF DF V 6–8 servings

Place all ingredients in the bowl of a food processor, and process until smooth. Taste, and adjust with additional salt, pepper, or spices.

TAHINI is a traditional Middle Eastern paste made from ground sesame seeds. Look for it where you find nut butters at the grocery store. Refrigerate tahini after opening.

Roasted Red Pepper Hummus

¼ cup raw almonds

1 (15-ounce) can garbanzo
beans, rinsed and drained

1 (7-ounce) jar roasted red bell
peppers, drained

1½ tablespoons extra-virgin
olive oil

1 tablespoon tahini

2 teaspoons smoked paprika

2 teaspoons paprika

1 tablespoon cider vinegar

Kosher or sea salt

Black pepper

Reminiscent of a Spanish sauce called romesco, this hummus has rich flavor and a beautiful reddish-orange color. Smoked paprika has a wonderful, lightly smoked flavor. If you like smoky flavors, you will love this spice and will find many other uses for it.

GF DF V 6–8 servings

1. In a food processor, finely chop almonds.

2. Add the beans, peppers, tahini, oil, spices, and vinegar, and process until smooth. Taste the hummus, then season with salt and pepper if needed.

Tzatziki Dip

1 mini or Persian cucumber (or ½ English cucumber)

1 (6-ounce) container plain Greek yogurt

1 tablespoon finely chopped red onion (or chives)

¼ teaspoon kosher or sea salt

Black pepper

1 tablespoon finely chopped fresh dill

1 ½ tablespoons finely chopped fresh mint

Zest of one lemon

Juice of half a lemon

2 garlic cloves, minced

1 tablespoon extra-virgin olive oil (optional)

This traditional Greek dip is tangy and fresh with the bright flavors of lemon, mint, dill, and garlic. The crunch comes from cucumbers and onion. Serve with raw vegetables, whole grain crackers, or whole wheat pita wedges. The recipe doubles easily for a larger group.

GF   **4 servings**

1. Quarter cucumber lengthwise, and slice out the seedy center. Slice quarters lengthwise into very thin strips, then chop across into very fine pieces.

2. Combine cucumber with the rest of the ingredients, and stir until combined. Cover and refrigerate for a few hours to allow the flavors to develop. Tzatziki will keep in the refrigerator for about 4 days.

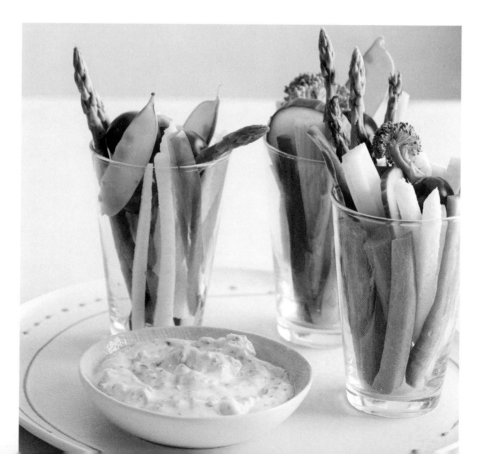

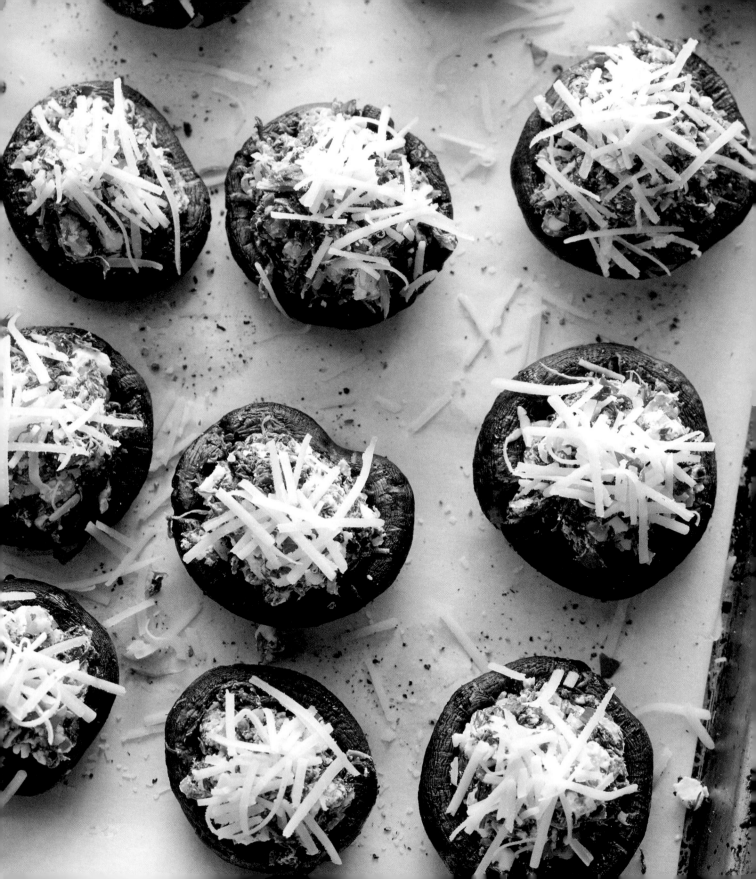

Spinach-Stuffed Portabellas

12 portabella mushroom caps or 24 large white mushrooms

2 tablespoons extra-virgin olive oil

½ teaspoon kosher or sea salt

¼ teaspoon coarse black pepper

1 (10-ounce) package frozen spinach, thawed

½ cup crumbled feta cheese

½ cup goat cheese

½ bunch green onions, chopped

2–3 cloves garlic, minced

½ cup minced fresh parsley

½ cup toasted walnuts, chopped

¼ cup grated Parmesan cheese

Popeye was right! Spinach is one of the world's healthiest foods. High in vitamins, spinach is one of the most nutrient-dense foods. One cup of these leafy greens contains far more than your daily requirements of vitamin K and vitamin A. It is an excellent source of more than 20 nutrients, including dietary fiber, calcium, and protein.

GF **12 mushrooms**

1. Preheat oven to 400°.

2. Remove the stems and gills from the mushroom tops. Place the mushroom caps onto a baking sheet stem-side down. Bake for 6–8 minutes or long enough for mushrooms to release their moisture and dry out.

3. Turn the caps stem side up, and brush each cap with olive oil. Season with pepper and salt. Set aside.

4. Reduce oven temperature to 350°.

5. Place a colander in a large bowl or the sink. Place the spinach in the colander, and press out all the water.

6. In another bowl, combine the spinach, cheeses, onion, garlic, parsley, and walnuts. Mix well. Divide the mixture between the caps. Sprinkle Parmesan cheese on top. Bake uncovered for about 15 minutes.

Food as Medicine

The mushroom family has powerful anti-inflammatory, cancer-preventing, and immune-boosting properties. Mushrooms are also full of minerals and are the best (and one of the only) vegetable source of vitamin D.

Shrimp Salad Spring Rolls

2 cups mixed greens

A few sprigs of mint, basil, or cilantro (optional)

½ cup shredded carrots

½ cup julienned cucumber, seeds removed

½ cup julienned mango

4 spring roll rice paper wrappers

8–12 medium cooked shrimp

½ cup Coconut Curry Dipping Sauce (page 177)

Dr. Amen Favorite

The fresh flavors and vibrant colors of the julienned vegetables wrapped in translucent rice paper wrappers make for an eye appealing starter to any meal. The original version of these rolls appeared in *The Omni Diet* by Tana Amen, B.S.N., R.N.   **GF DF   4–6 rolls**

1. Slice or julienne the greens, vegetables, and fruit.

2. Fill a medium or large bowl with warm water in which you can easily submerge the rice paper wrappers without breaking them. Dip a wrapper into the water for a few seconds just to wet. Shake excess water back in the bowl. (The rice paper will still seem stiff but will soften as you work with the rest of the ingredients. If you submerge in water longer, they will become too soft.)

3. Place ⅓–½ cup of mixed greens on top of the wrapper. Place 2 shrimp in the center of the greens. Follow with a few tablespoons of the carrot, cucumber, and mango lined up nicely on top of the shrimp and greens.

4. Roll the wrappers, folding the edge closest to you over the filling first, then folding in the two sides, and rolling toward the outside edge.

5. Allow the spring rolls to sit a couple of minutes before serving so that the paper can adhere to itself. If you'd like to prepare ahead, place the spring rolls on a sheet pan or plate lined with parchment paper and cover with plastic wrap to keep them moist.

> **TIP**   If the first wrapper tears or has a hole, simply prepare a second wrapper and double your spring roll.

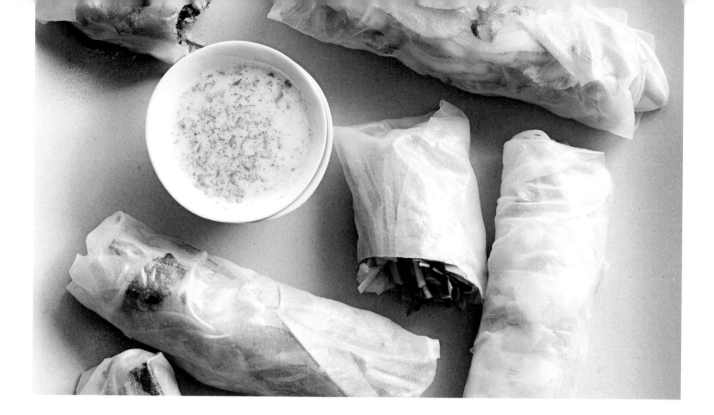

Coconut Curry Dipping Sauce

½ cup coconut milk

1 teaspoon raw honey

1 teaspoon toasted sesame oil

1 teaspoon minced fresh cilantro

½ teaspoon lime juice

½ teaspoon rice wine vinegar

¼–½ teaspoon curry powder

⅛ teaspoon cinnamon

⅛ teaspoon turmeric

Kosher or sea salt

Black pepper

A perfect companion to spring rolls or a stir fry, this sauce is like the icing on a dish—but good for you!

 ½ cup

In a small bowl, whisk all ingredients together. The mixture will be thin.

Avocado Ceviche

2 beefsteak tomatoes, diced

1 white onion, diced

½ cup fresh cilantro

2 tablespoons chili powder

Juice of 1 lemon

Juice of 1 lime

1 tablespoon kosher or sea salt

2 avocados, shaved into curls

This dish is an alternative to a fish ceviche but created in a similar manner: fresh herbs, vegetables, and citrus. Avocado ceviche is a perfect light snack to enjoy over greens, with baked tortilla chips (page 166) or as a filling for tacos or wraps. **GF DF V** **4 servings**

1. In a food processor, place the tomato, onion, cilantro, chili powder, juices, and salt. Pulse a few times. Mixture should be salsa-like in consistency to create the best ceviche.

2. To create an avocado curl, cut an avocado in half, remove the pit, and then using a spoon or a melon baller, curl out pieces of avocado that are about ¼-inch thick.

3. Remove the mixture from the food processor. Add the avocado curls. Fold together, then refrigerate. The best flavor will result if you make this ahead and chill the ceviche for about 24 hours. It will keep in the refrigerator for up to 5 days.

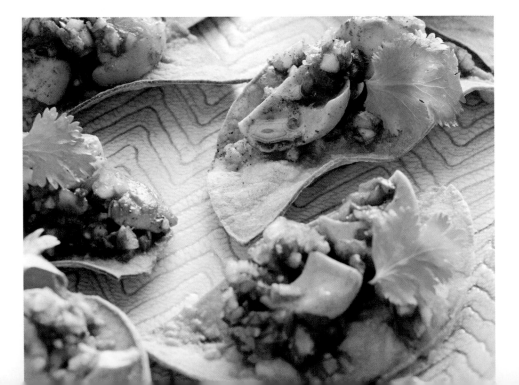

Spinach and Artichoke Dip

1 10-ounce box frozen spinach

12 ounces frozen or canned artichoke hearts

1 ½ tablespoon extra-virgin olive oil

¾ cup finely chopped onion

1 ½ teaspoons dried oregano (or 1 tablespoon fresh)

3 large garlic cloves, minced

5 ounces plain Greek yogurt

¾ cup grated Parmesan cheese

¾ teaspoon kosher or sea salt

¼ teaspoon black pepper

Savory and warm, this dip will be familiar but with a healthier profile. Serve with baked whole grain or rice chips or raw vegetables like red bell peppers. It could even work as a side dish. **GF** **4–6 servings**

1. Pre-heat oven to 350˚.

2. Cook frozen spinach according to package directions.

3. Place cooked spinach in a sieve and press out all water. Do the same with the artichoke hearts. Coarsely chop the spinach and artichokes.

4. In a medium pan, heat olive oil over medium-low heat. Add onion and oregano. Cook until soft. Add garlic, and cook 1 more minute while stirring.

5. Stir in artichokes, spinach, yogurt, and ½ cup of the Parmesan. Season with salt and pepper. For a creamier consistency, add a couple more tablespoons of Greek yogurt or vegan or organic mayonnaise.

6. Place dip in an oven-safe shallow dish and bake until heated through. Top with the remaining ¼ cup of Parmesan, and serve. If you want to brown the top, place under a hot broiler for 1 minute until cheese melts.

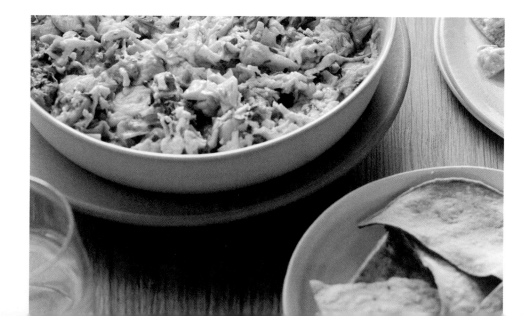

Homemade Granola Three Ways

Base

4 cups of toasted buckwheat groats or rolled oats

Blueberry peach

1 cup dried peaches

1 cup dried blueberries

⅓ cup raw agave or raw honey

1 teaspoon kosher or sea salt

1 cup apple juice

⅓ cup unsweetened shredded coconut

Pistachio crunch

1 cup dried apples

⅓ cup raw agave or raw honey

1 tablespoon coconut oil

1 teaspoon kosher or sea salt

2 tablespoons cinnamon

1 teaspoon nutmeg

½ cup raw pistachios

Superfood snack mix

1 cup gogi berries

⅓ cup raw agave or raw honey

2 tablespoons coconut oil

1 teaspoon pure vanilla extract

1 teaspoon kosher or sea salt

1 cup hemp seeds

Avoid the additives found in many store-bought granolas by making your own. Get creative with flavors you love! Use your favorite granola to create granola "bars" or yogurt parfaits (see page 245 for the Ginger Peach Parfait). The instructions are the same for each variety.

DF **4 servings**

1. Preheat the oven to 350°.

2. Soak dried fruit in fresh water that covers the top of the fruit for about 5 minutes. Strain off the rinse water, and then dice the dried fruit and set aside.

3. In a large mixing bowl, combine agave or honey, oil, salt, and spices. Whisk well. Add any liquid ingredients (juice or extract) and whisk again.

4. Add buckwheat or oats, nuts, or seeds to the liquid, and toss together until all parts of the granola are coated. Fold in fruits.

5. Place the granola mixture in a medium baking dish at least 3 inches deep. Bake the granola for 25 minutes, stirring occasionally. Bake 5 minutes more at a time if the mixture is not crunchy. The granola should be dry before removing it from the oven.

6. Remove from the oven and let cool. Store in an airtight container. The mixture should keep in the pantry for at least 3 weeks.

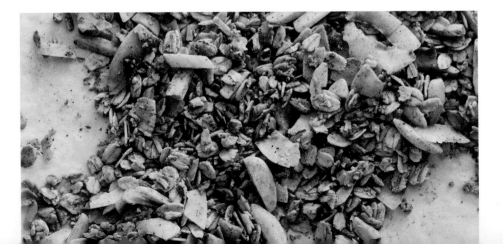

Blueberry Muffins

1 teaspoon extra-virgin olive oil

1 cup almond meal

2 teaspoons baking powder

2 teaspoons cinnamon

¼ teaspoon kosher or sea salt

4 large eggs

1 tablespoon unsweetened applesauce

1 tablespoon pure vanilla extract

1 cup frozen blueberries

Dr. Hyman Favorite

Typically, muffins are really miniature cakes packed with white sugar and flour. These muffins from Dr. Hyman's kitchen are absolutely guilt-free! Enjoy them any time as a snack or breakfast addition. The original version of these muffins appeared in *The Blood Sugar Solution Cookbook* by Mark Hyman, M.D.   **GF** **DF**   **6 muffins**

1. Preheat the oven to 350°.

2. Line a 6-cup nonstick muffin pan with baking cups, and lightly grease the cups with oil. (If you don't have a 6-cup pan, use a 12-cup pan and put a little water in each of the empty cups; this balances the baking area to help muffins cook evenly.)

3. In a large bowl, stir together the almond meal, baking powder, cinnamon, and salt.

4. In a separate small bowl, whisk together the eggs, applesauce, and vanilla.

5. Pour the wet ingredients into the dry ingredients, and mix until the batter is smooth. Fold in the blueberries.

6. Divide the batter evenly among the 6 muffin cups. Give the pan a few gentle taps on the counter to remove any air bubbles trapped in the batter.

7. Bake for 25–30 minutes. The muffins are done if a toothpick comes out clean when inserted into the center of a muffin. Let the muffins cool on a wire rack for 10 minutes before serving. Leftover muffins can be stored in the refrigerator for 2 days or in the freezer for up to 6 months.

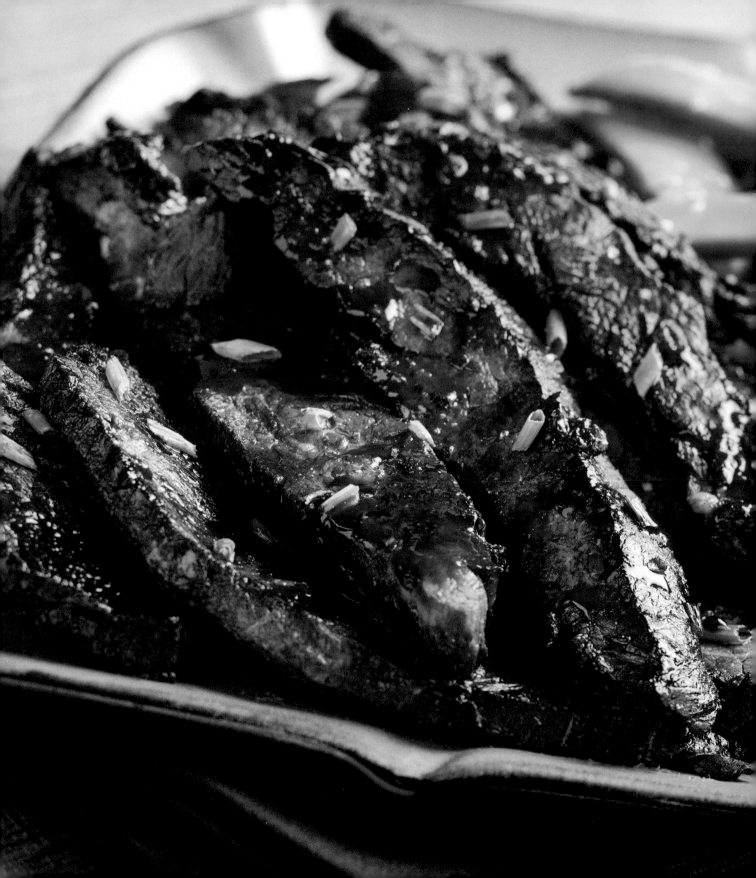

Fish, Chicken, and Beef

Coconut-Lime Shrimp Skewers

2 (15-ounce) cans coconut milk

½ cup lime juice (5–6 limes)

4 tablespoons wheat-free tamari or soy sauce

3 tablespoons toasted sesame oil

2 tablespoons ginger puree/paste

3 large garlic cloves, minced

⅛ teaspoon crushed red pepper (or liquid hot sauce)

1¼–1½ pounds large raw shrimp, peeled and deveined

Kosher or sea salt

Black pepper

Coconut milk and lime juice do double duty as a marinade and sauce for tropically inspired grilled shrimp. Use an outdoor grill, a grill pan, or the broiler for cooking. Serve with Chinese black "forbidden" rice or brown rice and roasted asparagus for striking color and flavor.

GF **DF** **4 servings**

1. Whisk together the coconut milk, lime juice, soy sauce, sesame oil, ginger, garlic, and red pepper flakes. Place half of the marinade in a bowl, dish, or sealable plastic bag and the other half in a small saucepan.

2. Add shrimp to the bowl with the marinade. Marinate shrimp at room temperature for 20–30 minutes. If using bamboo skewers, soak in water while shrimp are marinating.

3. Bring the marinade in the saucepan to a boil, then turn to low and simmer for a few minutes until thickened. Sauce will turn a golden color and reduce in volume.

4. Drain the marinade from the shrimp. Discard marinade. Skewer shrimp on metal or bamboo skewers between the tail and top end. Sprinkle with salt and pepper. Place shrimp on a hot grill. Cook just a few minutes, until they turn pink on each side. Timing will depend on the size of your shrimp. Serve with the sauce.

TIP If shrimp are frozen, submerge in the bag under cold water until thawed, then use.

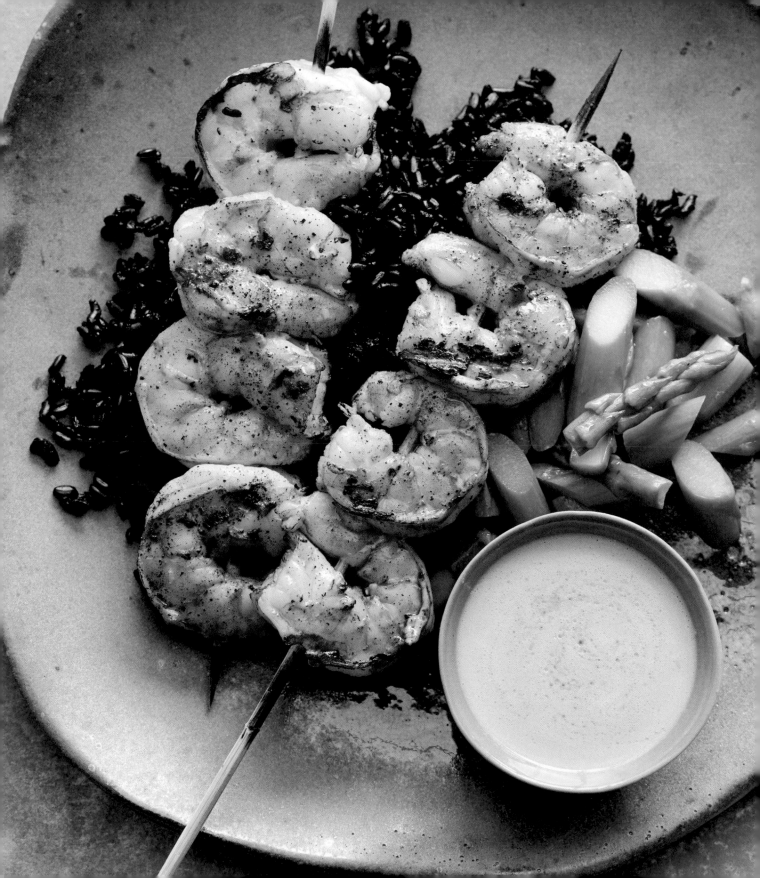

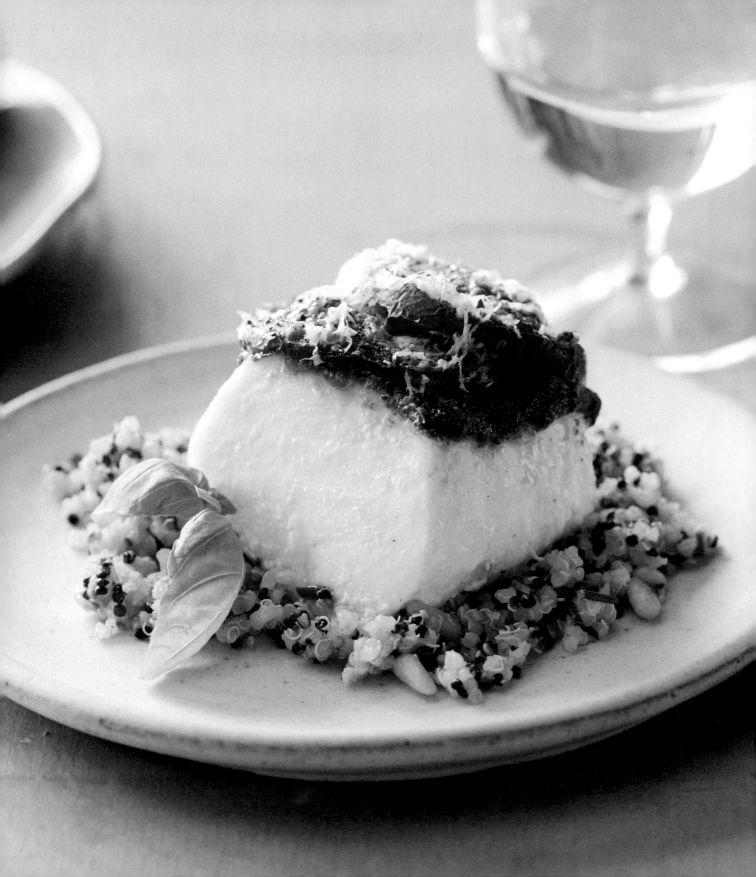

Roast Halibut with Pesto and Tomatoes

Pesto

1 cup fresh basil

1 cup extra-virgin olive oil

4 cloves garlic

1 teaspoon kosher
or sea salt

½ cup raw pistachios

Fish

1 teaspoon grape seed or
extra-virgin olive oil

1½ pounds of skinless
halibut, cut into 4 equal
portions

2 tomatoes, thinly sliced

Black pepper

3–4 tablespoons grated
Parmesan cheese (omit
for DF)

4 lemon wedges
(optional)

Roasting halibut is easy and will give you confidence for cooking fish. When buying fish, ask the fishmonger to skin it and cut it into equal portions to save you time. Plan for about 6 ounces per person. If halibut is not available, ask what firm white fish would be a good substitute. Serve with brown or wild rice and vegetables. **GF** **4 servings**

1. Put basil, oil, garlic, salt, and pistachios into a food processor. Pulse several times until blended well.

2. Preheat oven to 425°. Cover a rimmed baking sheet with foil. Brush with oil.

3. Place halibut filets on the foil. Spread with pesto, and top with a few overlapping slices of tomato. Sprinkle with pepper and Parmesan cheese.

4. Roast for 10–11 minutes (for fish that is 1¼-inch thick). Adjust your timing if the filets are thicker or thinner. Cheese will be melted and starting to brown, and fish will be just firm. When you cut into the filets, the fish will still be moist and just barely opaque. Serve with lemon wedges.

5. Serve over leftover quinoa or wild rice.

Easy Roast Salmon

4 (6-ounce) wild salmon filets, skinned

Kosher or sea salt

Black pepper

Granulated garlic powder (or your favorite spice blend)

4 teaspoons extra-virgin olive or grape seed oil

Sauce of your choice (optional)

This recipe will teach you how easy it is to enjoy salmon at home. This simple preparation lends itself to many sauces for different flavors such as barbecue, salsa, tzatziki, or pesto. Check the index for a list of Daniel Plan sauces. Ask the person at the fish counter to skin the filets for you to save time. **GF** **DF**   **4 servings**

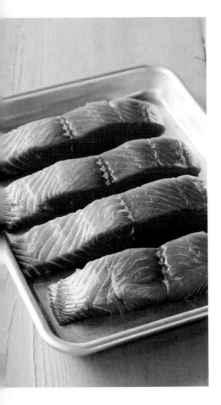

1. For best results, allow filets to stand unwrapped at room temperature for about 30 minutes to get the chill off before cooking.

2. Preheat oven to 425°.

3. On the skin side (the bottom side) of the filet, trim out any dark purple bloodline with a thin, sharp, flexible knife and discard. (The bloodline has a strong taste some people do not enjoy.) Turn filet over to the top side, and sprinkle with salt, pepper, and garlic. Drizzle oil over the top of each filet.

4. Over medium-high heat, heat an oven-safe pan large enough to hold all four filets without crowding them. When pan is hot, place the fish top side (seasoned side) down in the pan. You should hear it sizzle. This tells you the pan is hot enough. Sear salmon until you get a nice crust on the filet. It will take a few minutes. Watch your heat. You don't want the salmon to burn, but to get a good crust.

5. Turn filets over, move the pan to the hot oven, and roast for 2–4 minutes, depending on thickness. Remove from the oven and serve with your sauce or sides.

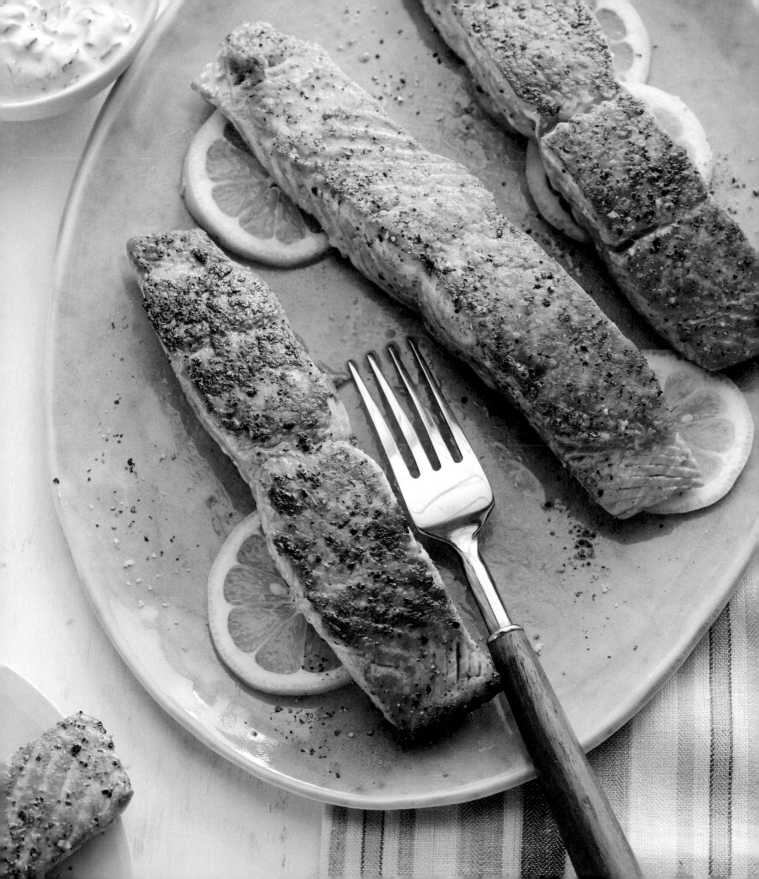

Crispy Baked Fish Sticks

1½ pounds sole, tilapia, or any low-mercury white fish

½ teaspoon extra-virgin olive oil

1½ cups whole wheat or gluten-free bread crumbs

½ teaspoon kosher or sea salt

½ teaspoon black pepper

1 teaspoon paprika

2 large eggs, beaten

Fish sticks are usually deep fried. This version uses fresh fish that is baked with olive oil. Create your own dipping sauce, such as Tartar Sauce (below) that lines up with The Daniel Plan principles.

DF **4 servings**

1. Preheat oven to 450°. Line a baking sheet with lightly greased aluminum foil or parchment paper. Set aside.

2. In a medium bowl, combine bread crumbs, salt, pepper, and paprika. Mix well. Slice fish into equal pieces about 1-inch wide. Gently submerge one piece of fish into beaten eggs to coat the entire surface of the fish. Immediately transfer fish to the bread crumb mixture. Coat with seasoned bread crumbs. Repeat with each piece of fish.

3. Spread breaded fish sticks across the baking sheet. Bake for 10–12 minutes, or until fish is completely cooked through. Remove from heat, and let sit for 3–5 minutes before serving.

Tartar Sauce

½ cup plain Greek yogurt

½ cup organic or vegan mayonnaise

2 medium dill pickles, finely chopped

¼ cup finely chopped red onion

2 teaspoons lemon juice

½ teaspoon granulated garlic powder

Black pepper

Omit sugars and additives, and most condiments will taste even better homemade. This sauce will dress up any fish with a little tang and zippiness.

GF **4 servings**

1. Thoroughly mix yogurt and mayonnaise in a small bowl.

2. Stir in remaining ingredients. Chill until ready to serve.

Baked Chicken Parmesan

4 boneless, skinless chicken breasts

1 cup whole wheat or gluten-free bread crumbs

¼ cup grated Parmesan cheese

1 teaspoon dried basil

½ teaspoon dried oregano

½ teaspoon granulated garlic powder

½ teaspoon onion powder

¼ teaspoon black pepper

2 tablespoons extra-virgin olive oil

½ cup shredded mozzarella cheese (omit for DF)

1 cup organic or Savory Spaghetti Sauce (page 107)

Traditionally made with chicken, veal, or eggplant, baked Parmesan dishes are loaded with Italian flavor. Serve with a side of roasted vegetables, such as broccoli with thyme, sautéed garlic spinach, or whole wheat or brown rice pasta.

4 servings

1. Preheat oven to 450˚.

2. Combine bread crumbs, Parmesan cheese, and spices in a bowl.

3. Lightly brush the chicken with olive oil. Dip chicken into breadcrumb mixture. Coat well. Place on baking sheet, and repeat with the remaining chicken. Lightly spray chicken with olive oil. Bake for 20 minutes.

4. Turn chicken over, and bake another 5 minutes. Spoon 1 tablespoon of spaghetti sauce on top of chicken. Cover chicken with 2 tablespoons mozzarella cheese. Bake another 5 minutes. Serve with a few tablespoons of spaghetti sauce.

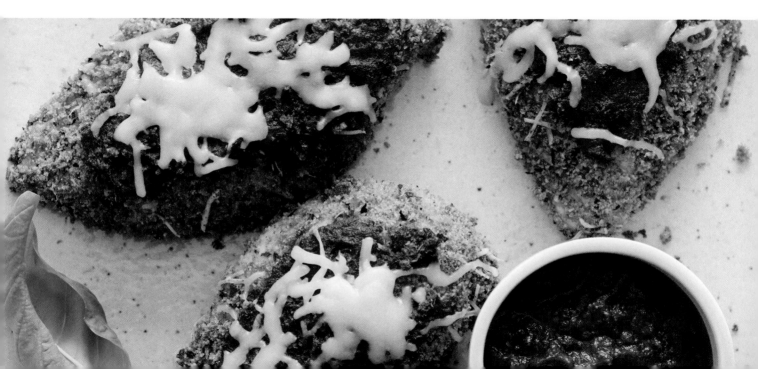

Grilled Rosemary-Lemon Chicken Kabobs

½ cup extra-virgin olive oil, plus extra for drizzling

¼ cup lemon juice

2 tablespoons finely chopped fresh rosemary

4 cloves garlic, finely chopped

1 tablespoon Dijon mustard

Kosher or sea salt

Black pepper

1½ pounds boneless, skinless chicken breast

1–2 red bell peppers

4 small zucchini

1 small Japanese eggplant (optional)

½ red onion (optional)

Cover Recipe

Tender pieces of grilled chicken with fresh flavors of rosemary and lemon make for a healthy and colorful dinner. Vary the vegetables according to your liking. Serve with brown rice and a tossed green salad. (While the cover photo shows the chicken and vegetables mixed on a skewer, they cook more evenly when skewered separately.)

GF **DF**   **4 servings**

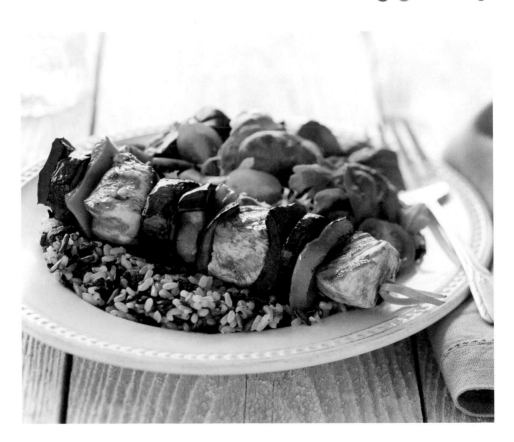

1. In a small bowl, whisk together oil, lemon juice, rosemary, garlic, and mustard. Add two good pinches of salt and a pinch of black pepper. Divide marinade into two portions, one as marinade for raw chicken and one to use as a sauce after grilling.

2. Cut chicken into large chunks, about 1½–2 inches in size. In a bowl or a sealable plastic bag, place chicken and half of the marinade. Stir or shake to coat chicken and allow to marinate 30 minutes at room temperature. Or marinate chicken in the refrigerator overnight for more flavor.

3. While chicken is marinating, cut peppers into 1½-inch chunks. Trim ends off zucchini, and cut into 1-inch pieces. Do the same with the eggplant and red onion.

4. Slide vegetables onto metal or bamboo skewers. Skewer the zucchini and eggplant through the sides so they lay flat on the grill. Drizzle vegetable skewers with a little olive oil and sprinkle with salt and pepper. Skewer the chicken pieces.

5. Preheat the grill. Oil the clean grates with a grill-safe spray or with a wad of folded paper towels dipped in a little oil. Use tongs to hold the paper towel wad while greasing the grates.

6. Grill chicken and vegetable skewers until chicken pieces are golden but not dry and vegetables are browned at the edges. If the vegetables get done more quickly, move them to a cooler part of the grill or place in a 200° oven to stay warm. Use the other half of the reserved marinade as a sauce to brush over the grilled skewers.

TIP   If you do not have a grill or weather does not permit, kabobs can be cooked under a preheated broiler. Use the second level down from the top rack. Turn the skewers half way through cooking.

IF USING BAMBOO SKEWERS, soak them in cold water for 20–30 minutes to help prevent them from burning.

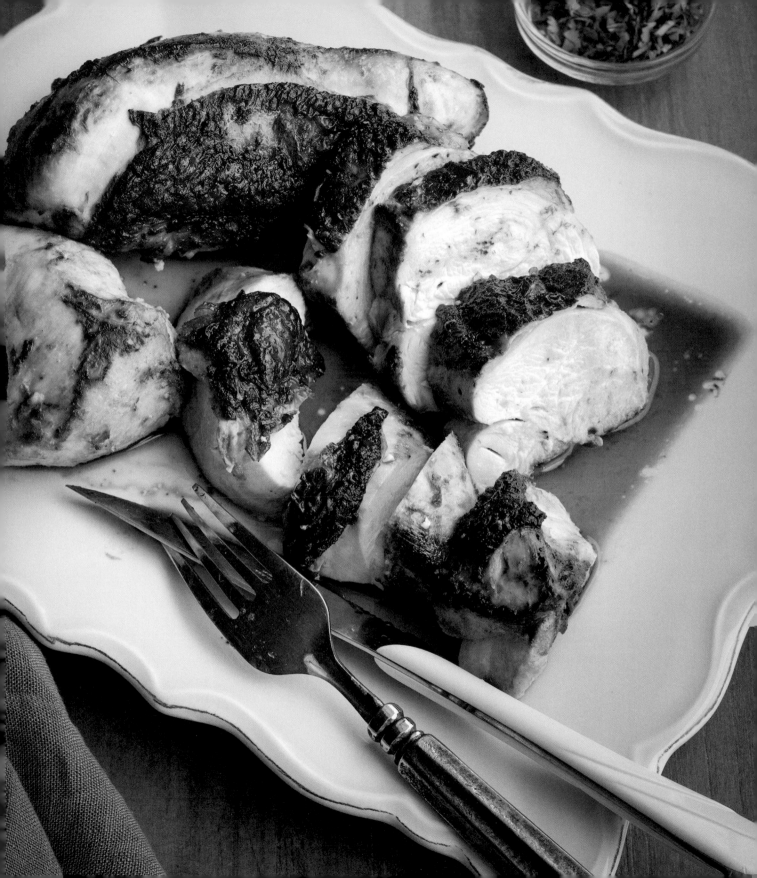

Simple Roasted Chicken Breasts

4 bone-in, skin-on chicken breasts

Kosher or sea salt

Black pepper

Granulated garlic powder

2 tablespoons olive, grape seed, or coconut oil

Bone-in chicken breast has great flavor and moisture because of the bone. From start to finish they take about 35 minutes. Roast an extra breast or two for chicken salad, sandwiches, or tacos. Leftover chicken is a handy staple to have in the refrigerator or freezer for future use. Serve simply with a squeeze of lemon juice and a drizzle of olive oil.

GF **DF**   **4 servings**

1. Preheat oven to 375°.

2. With a sharp, heavy knife or poultry shears, trim off the small rib bones on the side of each chicken breast and discard. Trim off extra fat, but leave most of the top skin on for searing and roasting.

3. Heat a large heavy pan, such as a cast iron skillet or stainless steel frying pan over medium heat for a few minutes. Add oil. Sprinkle chicken with salt, pepper, and garlic.

4. Place the chicken top side (skin side) down into the pan. The chicken should sizzle when it hits the pan. Sear until golden, then turn chicken breasts over and sear on bottom and side.

5. Place the pan directly into the oven for approximately 25 minutes. Exact roasting time will depend on the size of the chicken breasts. Chicken is done when a digital kitchen thermometer reads 165° when inserted into the thickest part without touching the bone.

6. Remove the skin and serve. Cool any extra chicken, then shred the meat to use for other meals. Extra chicken will keep 4 days refrigerated or 1 month frozen.

Oven-Fried Chicken

Extra-virgin olive oil

8 ounces plain Greek yogurt

1 tablespoon Dijon mustard

2–3 garlic cloves, minced

1 teaspoon dried basil

½ teaspoon kosher or sea salt

¼ teaspoon black pepper

¼–½ teaspoon hot sauce

2 cups organic corn flakes

4 tablespoons ground flaxseed

1½ pounds boneless, skinless chicken breasts

This crispy chicken provides a satisfying crunch, much like fried chicken, but without the grease and long, messy process. The crunch comes from organic cornflakes, flax meal, and a coating of spiced Greek yogurt. Enjoy whole with vegetables or sliced over salad greens with a homemade dressing.

GF **4 servings**

1. Preheat oven to 375°. Line a rimmed baking sheet with foil, and top with a wire rack. Oil the rack and foil.

2. In a medium bowl, stir together the yogurt, mustard, garlic, basil, salt, pepper, and hot sauce until smooth.

3. Place cornflakes into a sealable plastic bag, and crush them finely with a rolling pin, the flat side of a frying pan, or your hands. Add ground flaxseed and a sprinkle of salt and pepper to the cornflakes. Reseal the bag. Shake to mix. Pour into a pie plate or onto a sheet of waxed paper.

4. Put a dollop of the yogurt sauce onto each chicken breast, then spread to coat both sides. (Do not contaminate the yogurt sauce with raw chicken; you'll want the leftover sauce for serving.)

5. Nestle each chicken breast into the cornflake mix, and pat gently to create a solid coating. Coat both sides. Discard the unused crust mix.

6. Place the crusted chicken breasts on the wire rack. Bake for 18 minutes, until chicken feels firm and the crust is golden. If using a digital thermometer, internal temperature should reach 165°. Serve with extra yogurt sauce.

Chicken Veggie Stir-Fry

½ pound boneless, skinless chicken breasts, cut into 1-inch strips

2 cloves garlic, minced

1 tablespoon minced fresh ginger

1 jalapeno, seeded and minced

3 tablespoons wheat-free tamari or soy sauce

½ cup low-sodium chicken or vegetable broth, plus a few tablespoons extra

3 tablespoons cornstarch

1 tablespoon sesame oil

1 tablespoon coconut oil

2 cups small broccoli florets

1 cup corn

½ cup sliced water chestnuts, sliced

½ cup shredded carrots

½ cup bean sprouts

½ cup mushrooms, quartered

3 scallions, sliced diagonally

1 teaspoon sesame seeds

2 cups cooked brown rice

This is a crowd pleaser that's bursting with vegetables, fiber, and vitamins. This recipe also works well with lean trimmed beef, seafood, or turkey.

GF **DF** **4 servings**

1. In a medium bowl, mix the chicken strips, garlic, ginger, jalapeno, and 1 tablespoon of the soy sauce. Set aside.

2. In a small container, combine the remaining soy sauce, chicken broth, corn starch, and sesame oil. Place lid on container, and shake well. Set aside.

3. In a large sauté pan or wok, heat the coconut oil over high heat. Stir-fry chicken until tender and almost done, about 4–5 minutes.

4. Reduce heat to medium, add the vegetables and remaining soy sauce. Cook until the sauce thickens and the chicken is no longer pink in the center, about 4 more minutes. If the sauce becomes too thick, thin with a little chicken broth or water. Garnish with scallions and sesame seeds. Serve over brown rice.

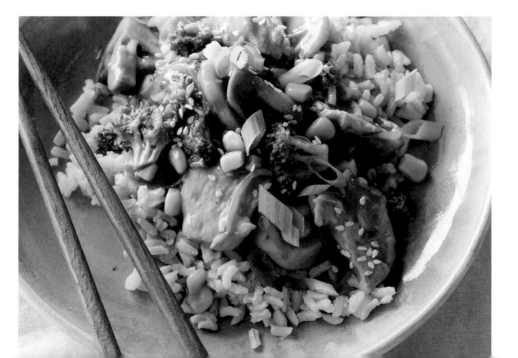

Asian-Style Curried Coconut Chicken

1 (14-ounce) can coconut milk

1 tablespoon sweet curry powder

1 tablespoon cornstarch

1 tablespoon lime juice

2 teaspoons raw honey

½ teaspoon kosher or sea salt

3 tablespoons coconut oil

1 pound boneless, skinless chicken breasts, cut into thin strips

1 red bell pepper, seeded and chopped

16–20 spears fresh asparagus, cut into 1-inch pieces

1 tablespoon grated fresh ginger

¼ cup fresh basil, cut into thin ribbons

4 tablespoons slivered almonds, toasted

3–4 cups cooked brown rice

3–4 tablespoons chopped green onions

Hot sauce (optional)

2 tablespoons coconut, toasted (optional)

Pastor Warren Family Favorite

Ethnic foods such as Thai, Japanese, and Indian often use fresh ingredients and healing spices, packing in the nutrients and flavor that make curries and stir fries a hit. This recipe combines some of the best ingredients from a number of Asian dishes. **GF** **DF** **4 servings**

1. In a small bowl, whisk together coconut milk, curry powder, cornstarch, lime juice, honey, and salt. Set aside.

2. Heat a wok or a large stainless steel sauté or frying pan over medium-high heat until a few drops of water evaporate immediately. Swirl 2 tablespoons of the coconut oil in the pan to coat. Add chicken strips, and cook 2–3 minutes on each side, until golden. Remove chicken from the pan, and keep warm.

3. Heat the remaining 1 tablespoon of coconut oil in same pan over medium-high heat. Add bell pepper, asparagus, and ginger; cook for 3–4 minutes. Stir often.

4. Whisk sauce, and add to the vegetables. Cook until sauce thickens, about 1–2 minutes. Stir in basil, chicken, and nuts. Serve over hot rice. Garnish with green onions, hot sauce, and coconut.

Chile Verde Chicken

Verde Sauce

3 cups low-sodium chicken broth

16 small canned or fresh tomatillos

2 jalapenos, seeded and halved

3 garlic cloves, peeled

1 large white onion, chopped

1 bunch cilantro (about 3 ounces)

4 tablespoons of lime juice

1 teaspoon cumin

Kosher or sea salt

Black pepper

Chicken

2 tablespoons extra-virgin olive oil

Kosher or sea salt

Black pepper

4 boneless, skinless chicken breasts

Dr. Hyman Favorite

Ingredients such as cilantro, jalapenos, cumin, and pepper have powerful healing effects on your body. And they make chicken taste wonderful! The original version of this chicken appeared in *The Blood Sugar Solution Cookbook* by Mark Hyman, M.D.   GF DF **4 servings**

1. In a medium pot over high heat, bring broth to a boil. Reduce heat to medium-low. Add the tomatillos, jalapenos, and garlic cloves. Simmer until the vegetables are soft, about 5 minutes. Cool slightly.

2. Transfer the contents of the pot to a blender. Add the onion, cilantro, lime juice, cumin, salt, and black pepper while the blender is running. Blend until smooth, about 2 minutes. Set aside.

3. Heat the oil in a large sauté pan over medium-high heat. Season the chicken generously with salt and pepper. Place in the hot pan. Cook until all the chicken is brown, about 3 minutes per side.

4. Reduce the heat to low, and add the blended verde sauce. Cover the pan, and simmer until the chicken is very tender, 20–25 minutes.

5. Shred the chicken with two forks, and serve in the verde sauce. Any leftover chicken can be refrigerated for up to 3 days.

Teriyaki Beef Stir-Fry

½ cup water

⅓ cup wheat-free tamari or soy sauce

2 drops liquid stevia extract

¼ cup fresh orange or pineapple juice

4 garlic cloves, minced

1 inch fresh ginger, peeled and cut into thin strips

1 pound flank steak, cut against the grain into thin strips

2 teaspoons coconut oil

4 cups broccoli florets

1 medium onion, chopped

1 tablespoon minced fresh ginger

1½ teaspoon cornstarch

2 cups brown rice

One of the most popular Asian meals that many of us enjoy is filled with broccoli. The broccoli florets absorb all the delicious flavors of the seasonings in the dish. Plus, broccoli is a health goldmine — you can never eat enough of it.

GF **DF**   **4 servings**

1. In a small bowl, combine the water, soy sauce, stevia, juice, garlic, and ginger strips. Pour ½ cup of it into a plastic bag; add beef. Seal bag, and turn to coat the beef. Refrigerate for at least 1 hour. Cover and refrigerate remaining marinade.

2. Remove steak from bag, and discard marinade. In a large nonstick skillet or wok, stir-fry beef in oil for 2–3 minutes or until no longer pink. Remove from pan but keep warm.

3. Add broccoli, onion, and minced ginger to pan; stir-fry for 4 minutes or until vegetables are tender.

4. Return beef to the pan. Whisk cornstarch and reserved marinade until smooth; stir into beef mixture. Bring to a boil; cook and stir until thickened, about 2 minutes. Serve over rice.

TIP   Marinate the steak overnight to save time the day of cooking.

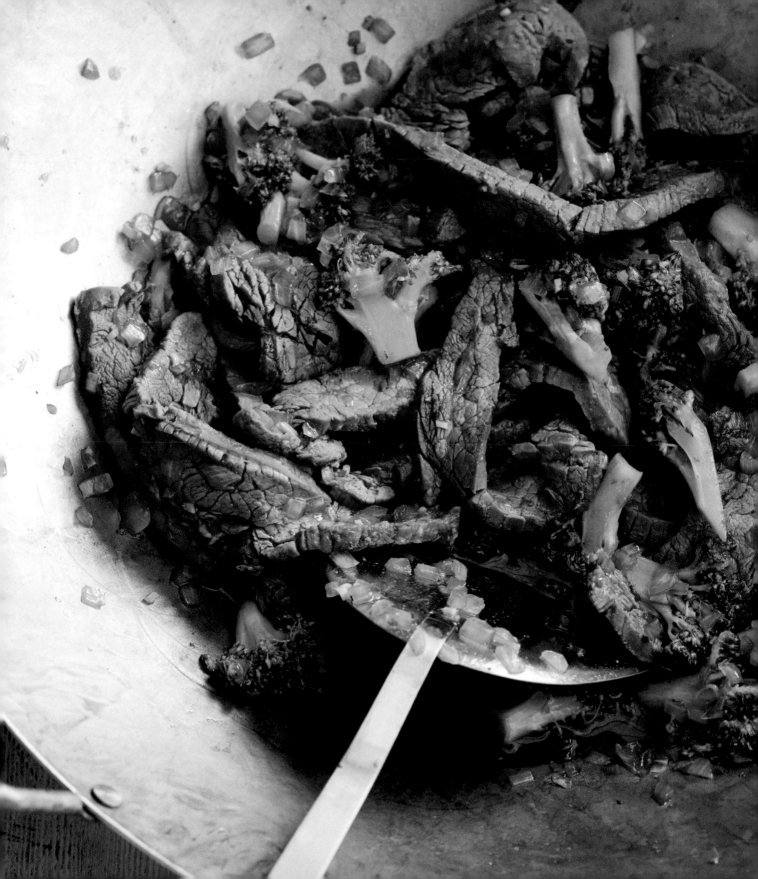

Pan-Seared Flank Steak

¾ cup low-sodium beef broth

¼ cup red wine vinegar

1 shallot (about 3 tablespoons)

3 tablespoons grape seed oil

4 garlic cloves

1 tablespoon fresh rosemary

1 tablespoon fresh cilantro

1 teaspoon Dijon mustard

1 teaspoon kosher or sea salt

½ teaspoon black pepper

1–2 pounds flank steak, trimmed

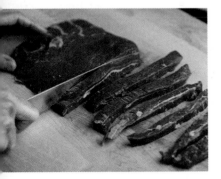

Dr. Amen Favorite

Flank steak is a good, lean cut that must be marinated for tenderness. Prep the night before to let the meat marinate several hours for incredible flavor. **GF** **DF** **4–6 servings**

1. In a food processor or blender, blend the broth, vinegar, shallot, 2 tablespoons of the grape seed oil, garlic, rosemary, cilantro, mustard, salt, and pepper.

2. Pour the marinade into a sealable plastic bag, and add the steak. Make sure the steak is completely covered with the marinade. Place the bag in a bowl then into the refrigerator. This steak is best if marinated for 2 to 24 hours. At the very least, marinate it for 30 minutes.

3. Preheat the oven to 400°, and set a rack in the center of the oven.

4. Heat the remaining 1 tablespoon of grape seed oil in an ovenproof roasting pan over high heat. Remove steak from marinade, reserving the marinade. Add steak to hot roasting pan, and sear on one side for about 1 minute. Turn and sear on the other side for another minute. Steak should be browned on both sides. If not, turn again and sear for another 30 seconds on both sides.

5. Place pan in the oven for 5–7 minutes for medium rare, 8–10 minutes for medium, 10–12 minutes for well done.

6. Remove steak from the oven, and place on a cutting board. Cover with foil and allow to rest for 7–10 minutes.

7. Pour reserved marinade into the roasting pan, and place back on stovetop. Turn heat on medium high, and bring marinade to a boil. Reduce heat to simmer.

8. Slice steak into thin slices and place on serving platter or plates. Drizzle marinade over the top.

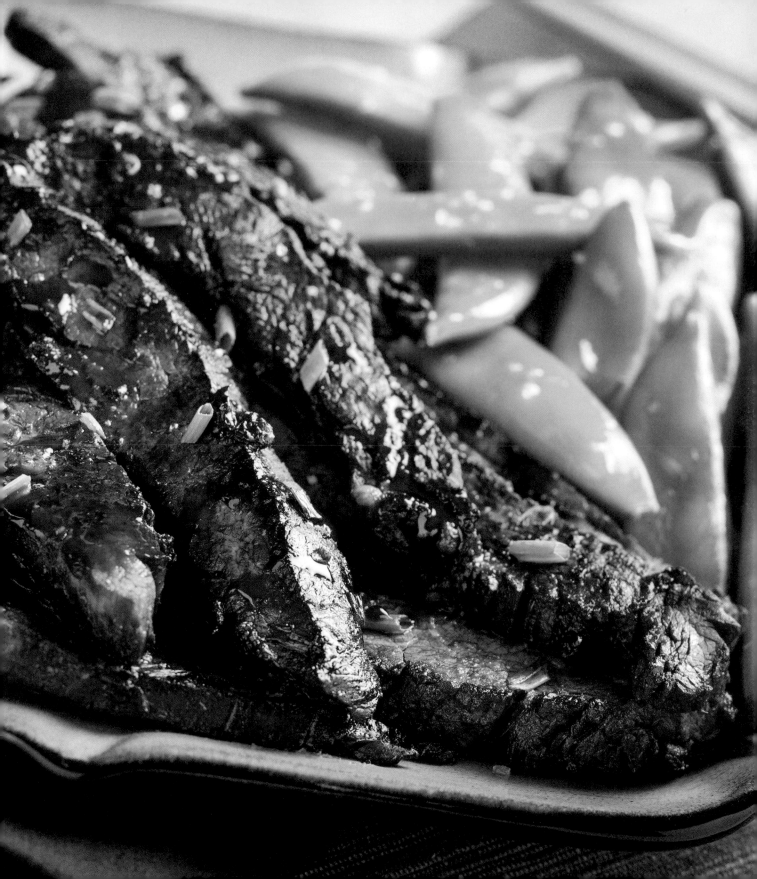

Mongolian Beef

½ cup wheat-free tamari or soy sauce

3 tablespoons balsamic or apple cider vinegar

1 tablespoon unsulphured molasses

2 tablespoons toasted sesame oil

½ cup orange juice

1 tablespoon raw honey

A few drops of Tabasco (or your favorite hot sauce)

8 ounces brown rice or buckwheat noodles

1¼ pound flank steak, cut against the grain into thin strips

⅓ cup cornstarch

4 tablespoons coconut oil

3 garlic cloves, minced

1 tablespoon grated fresh ginger

¼ – ½ teaspoon crushed red pepper

1 medium onion, halved and thinly sliced

3–4 tablespoons green onions, finely sliced

Pastor Warren Family Favorite

No MSG, no high fructose corn syrup, and no added salt! This entrée showcases an Asian-inspired classic with tons of flavor and nutrition.

GF **DF**   **4 servings**

1. Mix soy sauce, vinegar, molasses, sesame oil, orange juice, honey, and hot sauce in a small bowl.

2. Place sliced steak in a sealable plastic bag with cornstarch, and toss until well coated. Allow meat to stand for 10 minutes.

3. Bring a large pot of water to a boil, and cook noodles according to package directions. Keep hot.

4. Heat wok or a large stainless steel frying or sauté pan over medium-high heat until a few drops of water evaporate immediately when sprinkled on the surface. Swirl 1 tablespoon of the coconut oil in the pan to coat it. Add garlic and ginger; cook 30 seconds or until fragrant. Stir in sauce and boil for 3–4 minutes or until sauce thickens. Transfer sauce to a bowl; wipe pan clean.

5. Heat 1 tablespoon of the coconut oil in pan over medium-high heat. Add onion and stir-fry 2–3 minutes or until soft. Transfer onion to a bowl.

6. Heat 1 tablespoon of the coconut oil in pan over medium-high heat. Add half of the steak, and stir-fry 3–5 minutes or until meat is nicely browned. Remove from pan, and repeat with the remaining coconut oil and remaining steak. Stir in cooked onion and reserved sauce.

7. Place hot noodles in a shallow bowl or plate. Top with the steak and onions, and sprinkle with green onions. Add more hot sauce as desired.

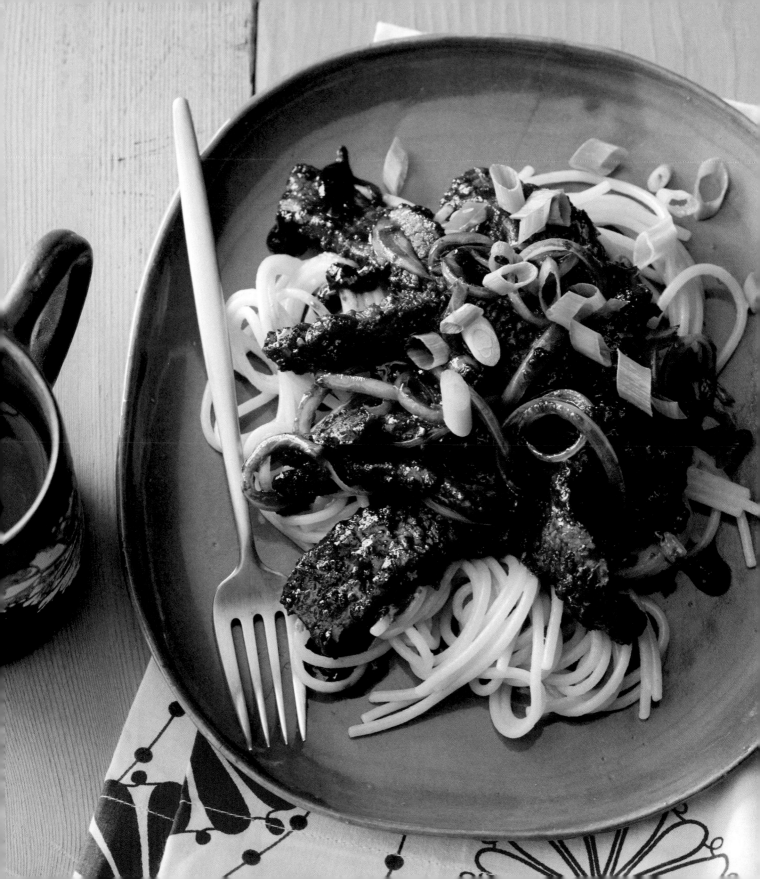

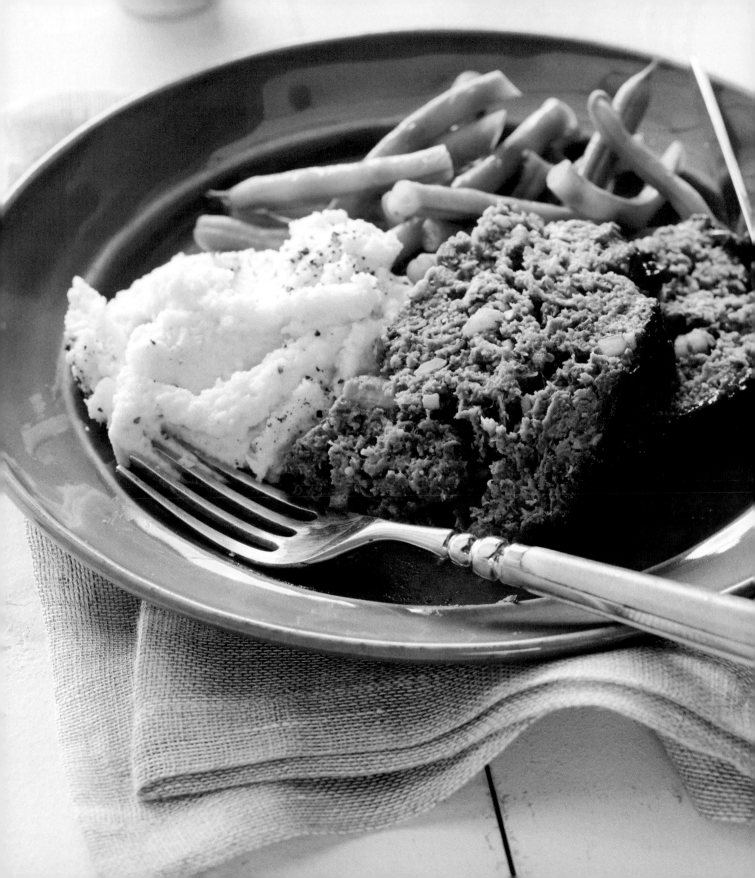

Classic Meatloaf

Meatloaf

Grape seed or extra-virgin olive oil

1 pound lean ground beef

1¼ cups toasted whole wheat or gluten-free bread crumbs

½ cup finely chopped Granny Smith apple

½ cup finely chopped onion

½ cup organic or Homemade Ketchup (page 226)

1 large egg

3 tablespoons chopped fresh Italian parsley

1 tablespoon coarse or whole grain Dijon mustard

1 teaspoon dried thyme (or 1 tablespoon fresh thyme)

½ teaspoon kosher or sea salt

¼ teaspoon black pepper

½ teaspoon granulated garlic powder

Glaze

½ cup organic or Homemade Ketchup (page 226)

1 tablespoon Worcestershire sauce (no HFCS)

¼ teaspoon black pepper

2–3 teaspoons chili powder

Pinch of ground chipotle powder or hot sauce (optional)

Apple adds flavor, moisture, and fiber to this modern, family-friendly meatloaf, but you will never know it's there. Leftovers make great sandwiches, or skip the bread and enjoy with a salad for lunch. Both meatloaf and bread crumbs freeze well. **DF** **4 servings**

1. Preheat the oven to 350°. Line a rimmed baking sheet with foil and coat lightly with oil.

2. In a large bowl, place the ground beef, bread crumbs, apple, onion, ketchup, egg, parsley, mustard, and seasonings. Mix gently but completely with your hands.

3. Gather the meatloaf mix into a ball, and place on the foil-lined baking sheet. With your hands, shape the meat into a smooth, long, oval loaf.

4. In a small bowl, mix the glaze ingredients. Brush half of the glaze on the meatloaf.

5. Bake for 35–45 minutes, or until meatloaf reaches 165° internally. Allow to rest for a few minutes, then slice and serve.

TIP   You may need to mix in an extra egg if the meat mixture feels dry.

FOR AN EXTRA RICH COATING   Brush the other half of the glaze over the meatloaf about halfway through baking.

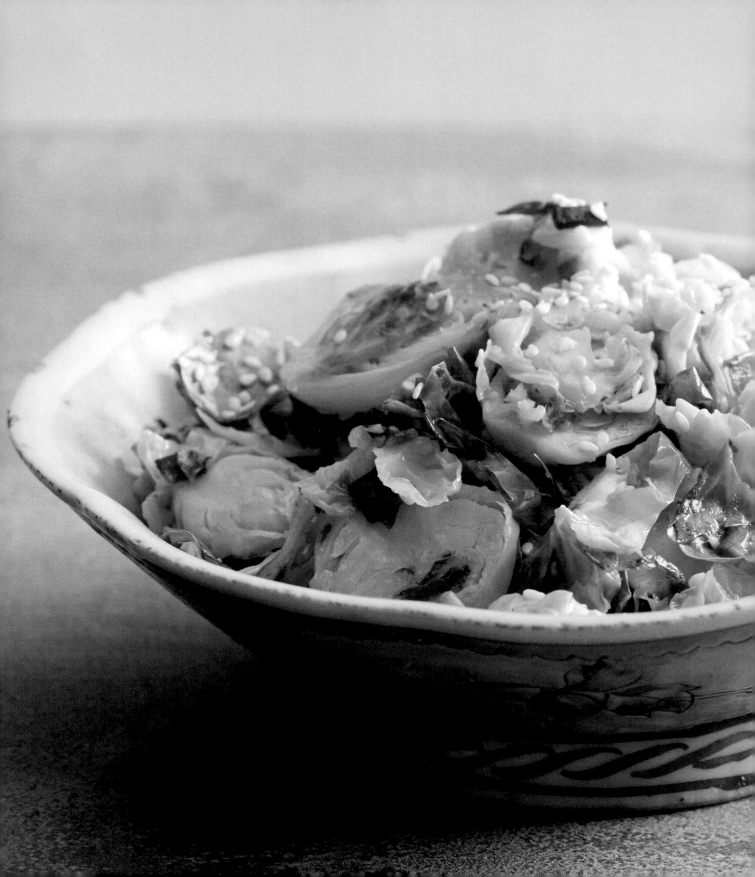

Side Dishes

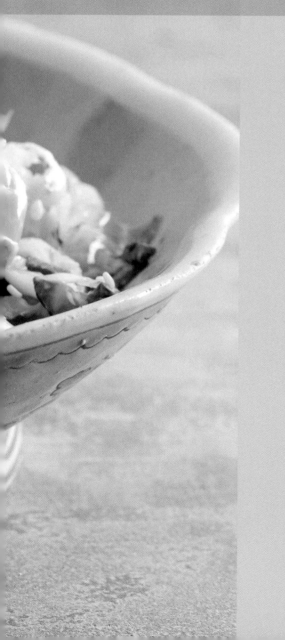

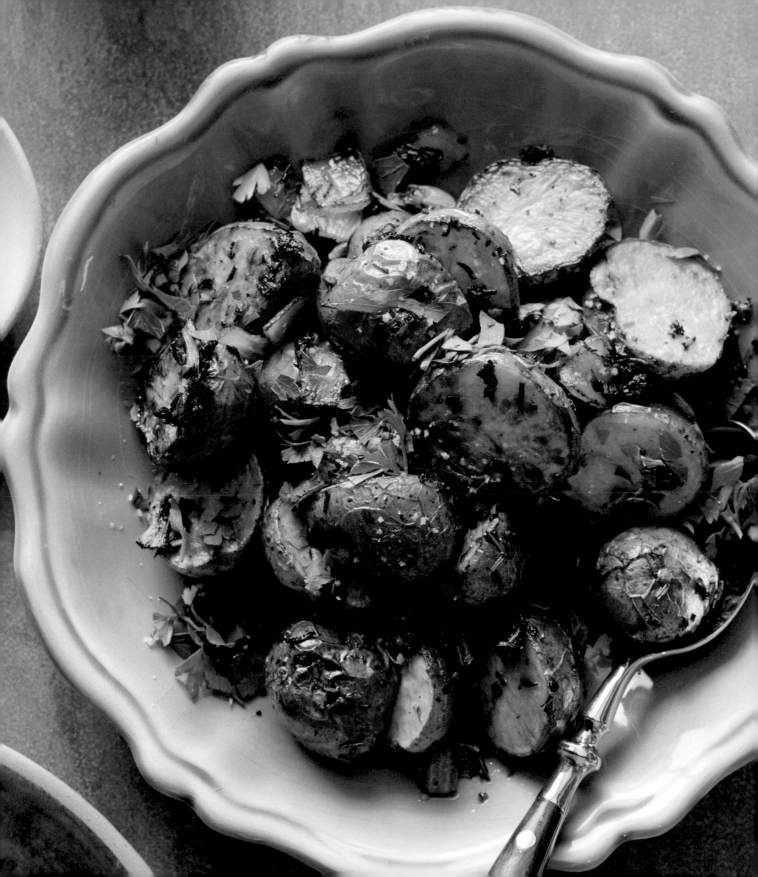

Roasted Rosemary Potatoes

10 – 12 small redskin potatoes, cut in half

½ cup diced sweet onion

3 tablespoons extra-virgin olive oil

1 tablespoon balsamic vinegar

¼ teaspoon Kosher or sea salt

¼ teaspoon black pepper

2 tablespoons chopped fresh rosemary

2 cloves garlic, minced

2 tablespoons chopped fresh parsley (optional)

eep the skins on potatoes to get additional vitamins and nutrients. You might also try sweet or purple potatoes as a variation.

GF DF V   **4 – 6 servings**

1. Preheat oven to 400°.

2. In a large bowl, toss all ingredients except the parsley until potatoes are lightly coated with olive oil mix.

3. Place potatoes on a baking sheet lined with parchment paper. Bake for 25 minutes. Remove potatoes from oven and gently toss, turning the potatoes over as needed. Bake for another 25 minutes or until potatoes are golden and tender. Sprinkle with the fresh parsley and serve.

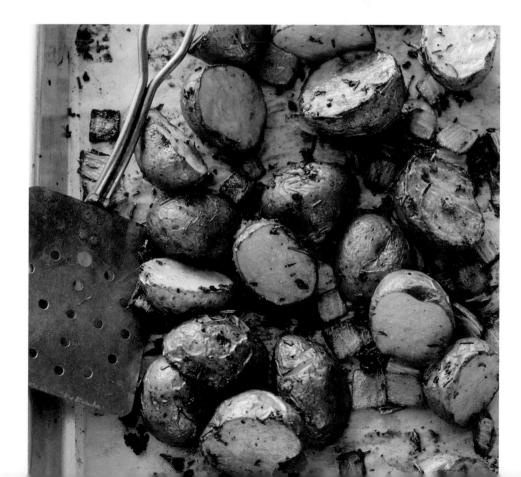

Faux Mashed Potatoes ("Creamed" Cauliflower)

2¼–2½ pounds white cauliflower (1 very large head)

3 tablespoons extra-virgin olive oil

1 large leek

2–3 teaspoons fresh thyme (or 1 teaspoon dried)

3 large garlic cloves, minced

½ cup grated Parmesan cheese

¼ cup sour cream

Kosher or sea salt

Black pepper

This creamy side dish may look like classic mashed potatoes, but it is made from steamed cauliflower pureed with heart-healthy olive oil, aromatic leek, fresh thyme, garlic, and Parmesan. **GF** **4 servings**

1. Cut the core out of the cauliflower head. Break the rest into small florets, trimming off any large stems. You should have about 8–9 cups. Bring several inches of water to a boil in a steamer. Add cauliflower, cover, and steam 13–15 minutes or until very soft. Drain water, and place cauliflower back in the pan to stay hot.

2. Trim off tough green top and root end of the leek. Use the white and pale green part only. Cut leek in half lengthwise, and run under cold water to remove sand and dirt. Cut the halves crosswise into thin slices.

3. Heat 1 tablespoon of the olive oil in a large sauté or frying pan over medium heat. Slowly cook leek with thyme over medium-low to medium heat until soft. Do not brown. Add garlic, and cook 1 more minute. Sprinkle with salt and pepper.

4. Add hot cauliflower and leek mixture to the bowl of a food processor. Add the Parmesan, the remaining 2 tablespoons olive oil, and sour cream. Puree until smooth and creamy. Taste, and add salt and pepper as needed.

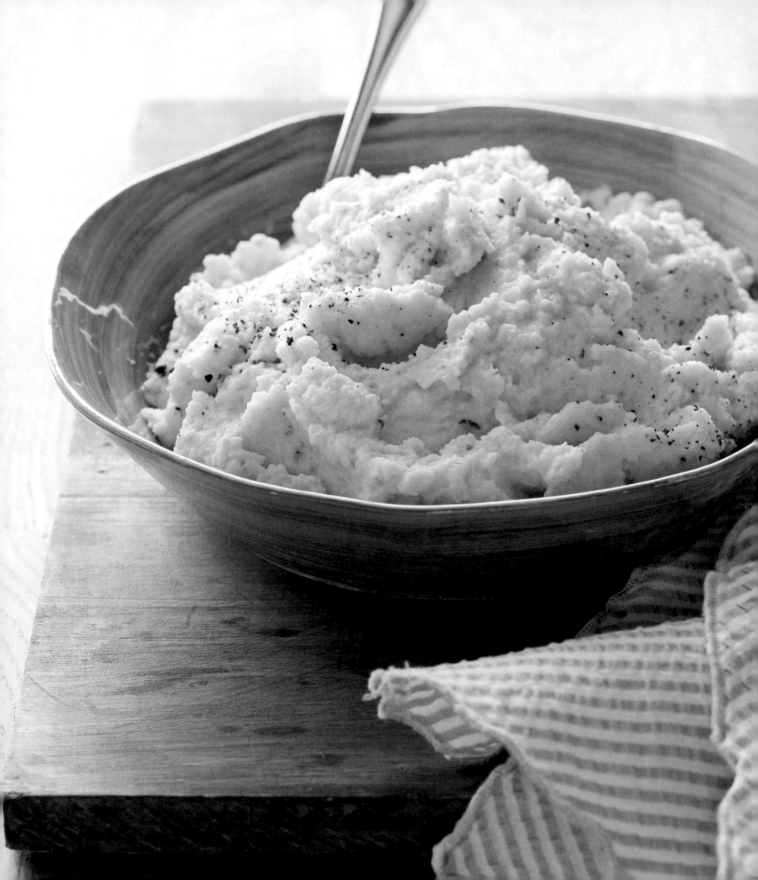

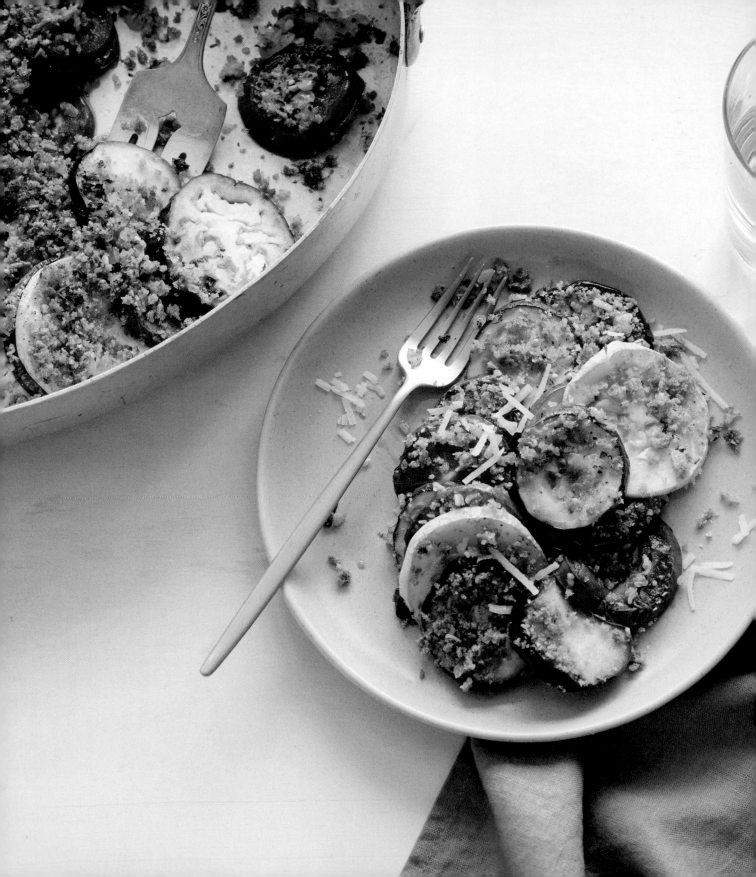

Vegetable Gratin

3 tablespoons extra-virgin olive oil

2 large zucchini, thinly sliced

1 yellow summer squash, thinly sliced

1½ pounds (about 7) Roma tomatoes, thinly sliced

½ small, thin eggplant, thinly sliced

¾ cup finely chopped onion

3 large garlic cloves, minced

Kosher salt

Black pepper

1 generous tablespoon minced fresh thyme

⅓ cup whole wheat or gluten-free bread crumbs, toasted

⅓ cup grated Parmesan cheese

A traditional dish from the south of France, this vegetable casserole is topped with bread crumbs and cheese for a crunchy, golden top. For squash, use a combination of green and yellow zucchini or summer squash. Slice vegetables to similar sizes for the best presentation.

6 servings

1. Preheat oven to 400°. Lightly oil a 9 × 13 oval or rectangular baking dish.

2. Layer the sliced squash, tomatoes, and eggplant in overlapping layers in the baking dish, alternating the colors, fitting them in the best you can.

3. In a sauté or frying pan, heat 1 tablespoon of the olive oil over medium heat. Add onion and cook until soft, stirring occasionally. Add garlic and cook 1 more minute. Stir in thyme, and remove pan from the heat. Distribute the onion mixture over the top of the vegetables. Sprinkle with salt and pepper.

4. Place bread crumbs and Parmesan in a small bowl with the remaining 2 tablespoons of olive oil, and mix with a fork until well blended. Sprinkle topping evenly over the vegetables. Place dish in the oven, and bake for 25–30 minutes or until vegetables are tender and crust is golden.

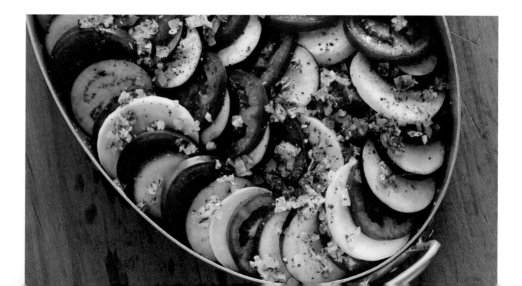

BBQ Yams

16 ounces tomato paste

2 tablespoons chili powder

1 tablespoon chipotle powder (optional)

1 tablespoon granulated garlic powder

2 tablespoons raw agave

1 teaspoon kosher or sea salt

2 medium yams

Imagine soft and sweet yams with a smoky, spicy barbecue sauce. This dish is simple but perfect to take along to potlucks, game nights, and neighborhood dinners. We recommend making a double batch as they save nicely all week long. **GF** **DF** **V** **4 servings**

1. Preheat the oven to 375°.

2. In a small mixing bowl, combine tomato paste, chili powder, chipotle powder, salt, garlic, agave, and salt. Whisk well or blend with an immersion blender. Transfer to a saucepan, and heat on low, stirring constantly for 4–5 minutes, until the mixture starts to boil and the color appears darker. Remove from heat, and set aside.

3. Rinse the yams well, but leave the skins on. Cut the yams lengthwise in half, then cut each section into ½-inch medallions.

4. In a medium mixing bowl, toss the yams and BBQ sauce until the yams are coated.

5. Line a baking sheet with parchment paper. Arrange the yams on top of the sheet. Bake for 35 minutes or until corners start to brown and crisp.

6. Remove from the oven, and let cool for 15 minutes. These yams may also be stored for up to 5 days in the refrigerator. They make a great filling for a taco shell or Napa cabbage leaf.

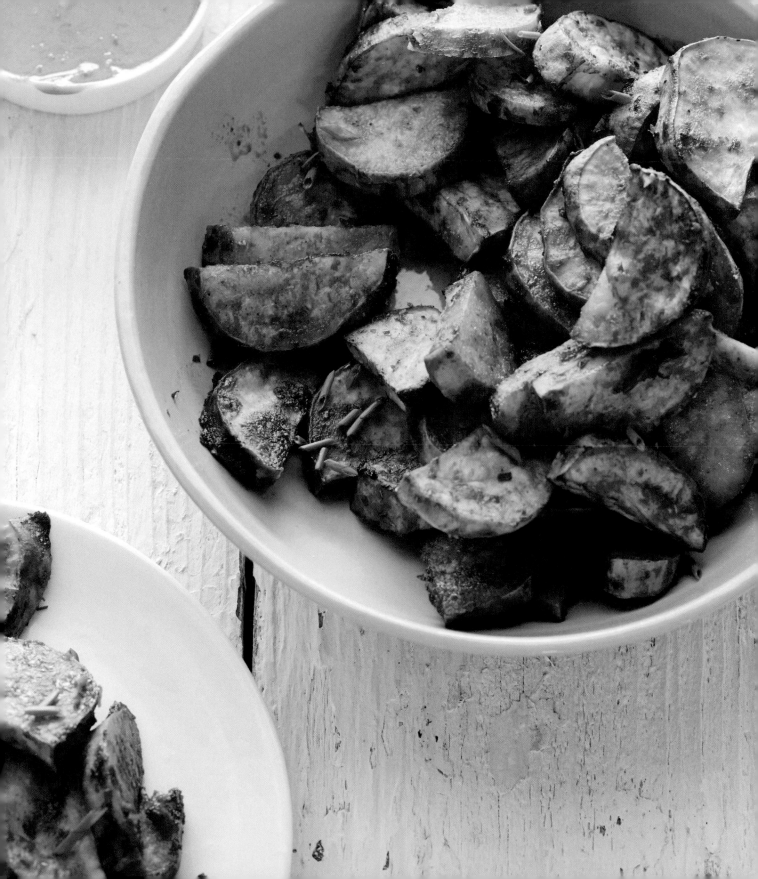

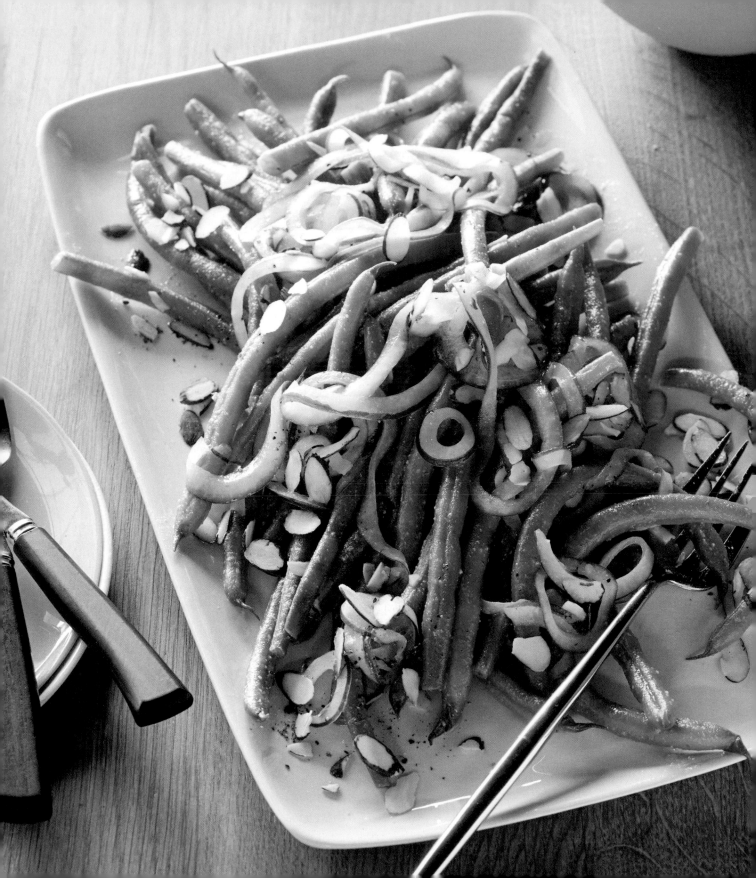

Miso Green Beans

Dressing

2 tablespoons white miso paste

1½ cups extra-virgin olive oil

2 cloves garlic, minced

2 inches green onion bulb (remove the green parts but save for garnish)

Beans

6 cups fresh green beans

1 cup marinated onions (optional)

1 cup sliced almonds or ½ cup diced walnuts (optional)

Miso is a great alternative to butter. It is naturally salty and creamy, so it's perfect for making a rich and creamy dressing without dairy, as we did for this simple dish. Use the dressing throughout the week with salads and other fresh vegetable dishes.

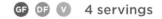 **4 servings**

1. Put the miso, oil, garlic, and onion in a blender. Combine until the mixture is smooth. Pour the dressing in a jar or other container.

2. Cut off the stems and harder tips from the green beans. Slice them in half if you prefer.

3. Fill a medium pot with water, place a steamer basket inside the pot, and fill with green beans. Cover pot, and cook over medium heat for 10 minutes. Remove the green beans while they are still firm but soft enough to easily bite through.

4. In a medium mixing bowl, toss the green beans with ½ cup of the dressing. Add optional toppings, and serve warm.

Food as Medicine

Green beans are a rich source of antioxidants, making them a great resource for cardiovascular health.

Emerald Broccoli

2 cups water

6 cups broccoli florets

1 cup organic or
homemade pesto
(page 187)

1 teaspoon kosher
or sea salt

2 tablespoons crushed red
pepper (optional)

1 lemon wedge

This is a simple beginner dish that makes a great side or even a meal served over 1 cup of brown rice or brown rice pasta. This broccoli also works nicely as a topping for Zucchini Pasta (see page 113).

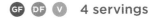 **4 servings**

1. Pour water into a medium pot with a steamer basket inside. Steam the broccoli for 6 minutes. Cover and let sit for 6 minutes. The broccoli should be an emerald green and still somewhat firm.

2. Remove the broccoli from the pot. In a medium bowl, toss the broccoli with pesto and salt while still hot. Sprinkle with red pepper flakes and a spritz of lemon. This dish will save for an additional 3 days in the refrigerator and is also delicious as a cold side salad.

Food as Medicine

Broccoli is rich in fiber, vitamins, and minerals, including folate and magnesium. Broccoli also contains powerful phytonutrients, which are healing plant compounds that help reduce the risk of cancer and boost your detoxification capacity. And broccoli has very little ability to raise your blood sugar.

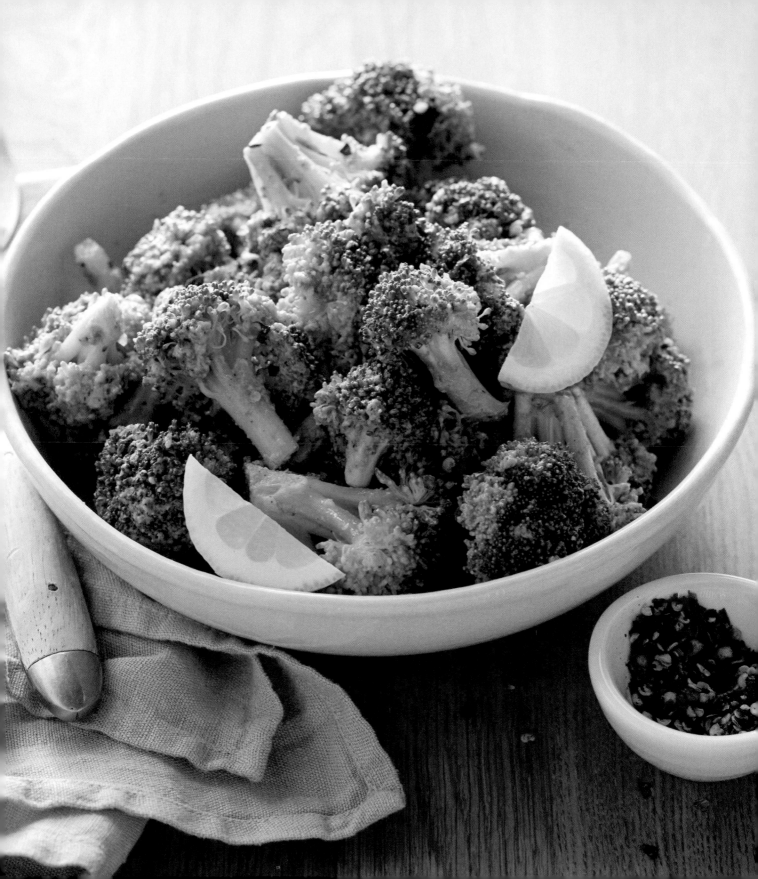

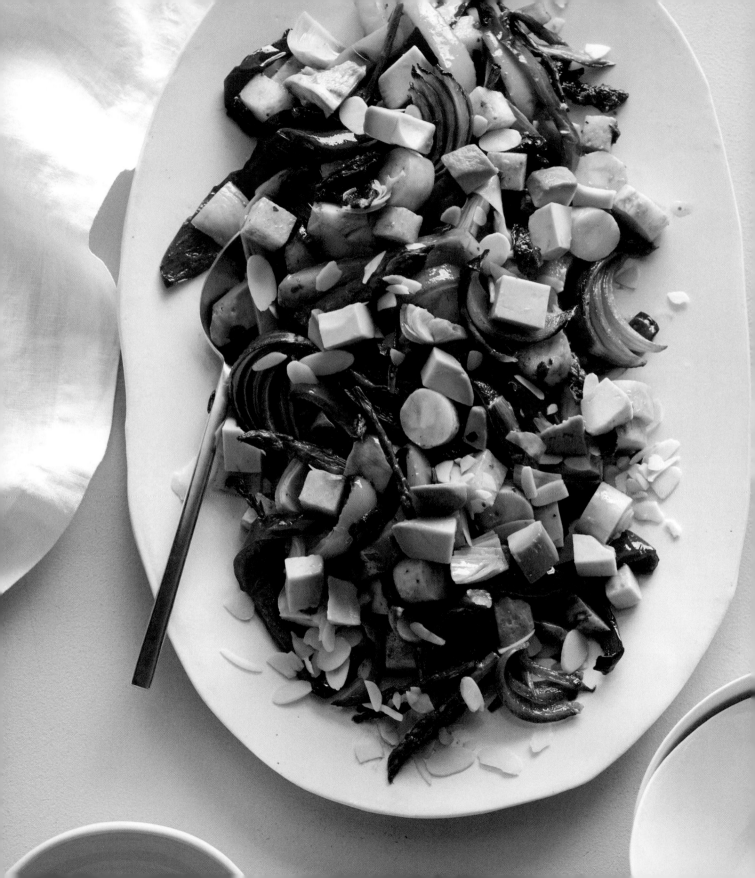

Roasted Vegetables

2 tablespoons grape
seed oil

2 red bell peppers, thinly
sliced

2 yellow bell peppers,
thinly sliced

½ red onion, sliced

2 cups asparagus tips

Kosher or sea salt

Black pepper

1 cup diced jicama

1 cup hearts of palm,
diced

1 cup sun-dried tomatoes,
sliced

1 cup artichoke hearts,
diced (optional)

½ cup extra-virgin olive oil

2 tablespoons balsamic
vinegar

1 tablespoon red wine
vinegar

1 tablespoon Dijon
mustard

1 garlic clove, minced

1 teaspoon raw honey
(optional)

½ avocado, diced

¼ cup slivered raw
almonds

Dr. Amen Favorite

Roasting brings out the natural flavor and sweetness of vegetables. Experiment by roasting a variety of vegetables to see how you can transform raw versions into a delicious, healthy side dish. The original version of this side dish appeared in *The Omni Diet* by Tana Amen, B.S.N., R.N.

GF DF **6 servings**

1. Preheat oven to 375°.

2. Lightly oil a large baking sheet. Spread peppers, onions, and asparagus on baking sheet and brush with the grape seed oil on both sides. Sprinkle with sea salt and pepper.

3. Bake for 30–40 minutes, or until vegetables are tender. Turn vegetables halfway through cooking time. Remove from oven, and allow to cool for at least 15 minutes.

4. In a large salad bowl, mix jicama, hearts of palm, tomatoes, and artichokes.

5. In a small bowl, combine olive oil, vinegars, mustard, garlic, and honey. Whisk well.

6. Combine roasted vegetables with raw vegetables. Add half of dressing, and toss well. Continue adding dressing and tossing until salad is lightly coated with dressing but not dripping.

7. Sprinkle avocado and almonds over the top.

> **TIP** Top this dish with roasted chicken (page 195)
> or pan-seared flank steak (page 202).

Asian-Style Brussels Sprouts

10–12 Brussels sprouts, cut into thin strips

1 tablespoon sesame oil

2 tablespoons diced turkey bacon

2 teaspoons minced fresh ginger

2 garlic cloves, minced

1 teaspoon sesame seeds

¼ teaspoon kosher or sea salt

Remember when your mom said to eat all your Brussels sprouts? Well, there is a very good reason. Brussels sprouts are especially high in vitamin K, which promotes healthy bones, prevents calcification of the body's tissues, serves as an antioxidant and anti-inflammatory agent, and is essential for proper brain and nerve function. This recipe will make you a believer and a fan of Brussels sprouts.

GF DF 4 servings

1. Warm sesame oil in pan over medium heat. Sauté turkey bacon, ginger, and garlic for 1 minute.

2. Add Brussels sprouts, and sauté till tender, about 3 minutes. Do not overcook or sprouts will get mushy. Season with sesame seeds and salt. Serve immediately.

Sweet Potato Fries

4 cups sweet potatoes,
cut into 4-inch sticks

4 tablespoons coconut oil,
melted

1 tablespoon chili-garlic
salt

Cut the sweet potatoes yourself, or defer to a bag of fresh frozen sweet potato pieces or sticks, which can often be found without preservatives. Serve these fries with Homemade Ketchup (page 226) or mustard. **GF** **DF** **V** **4 servings**

1. Preheat oven to 400°.

2. In a large mixing bowl, toss sweet potato sticks with the chili-garlic salt and coconut oil until all sticks are coated.

3. Line a baking sheet with parchment paper. Arrange the sweet potatoes on the baking sheet. Bake for 30–40 minutes, until crispy on the outside. Toss and rotate the fries about halfway through to make sure they cook evenly.

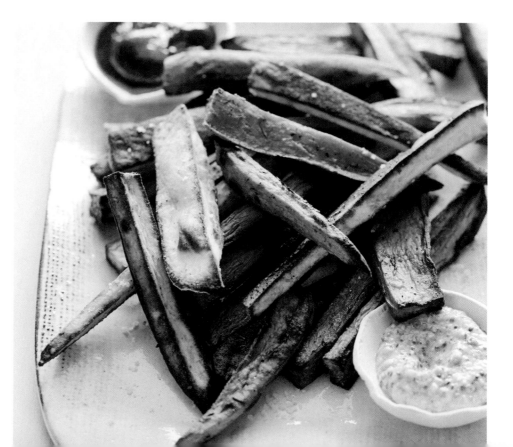

Homemade Ketchup

1 cup dried sun-dried tomatoes, soaked with water

2 tablespoons extra-virgin olive oil

2 tablespoons apple cider vinegar

1 tablespoon raw honey

1 teaspoon kosher or sea salt

Once you know how to make your own and see how easy it is, you'll have no problem keeping homemade ketchup on hand for any meal.

GF **DF** **1¼ cup**

Place all the ingredients into a food processor. Process into a thick paste. Use a spatula to scrape sides, and repeat the process one or two times. Remove the ketchup from the food processor, and refrigerate until ready for use. This homemade ketchup will keep for up to 7 days in the refrigerator.

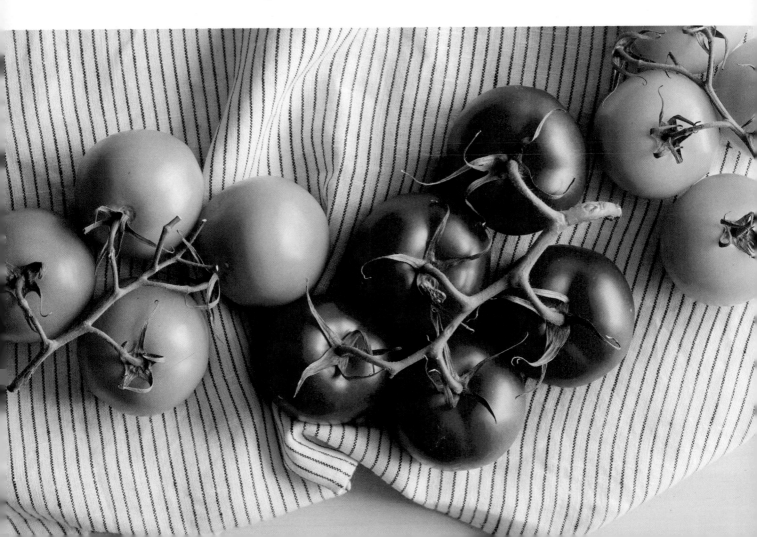

Cornbread with Honey Butter

Cornbread

1 (16-ounce) package gluten-free cornbread mix (e.g., Bob's Red Mill)

4 tablespoons ground gold flax seed

1 tablespoon baking powder

1 teaspoon baking soda

1 teaspoon kosher or sea salt

2½ cups water or almond milk

⅓ cup raw honey

4 tablespoons applesauce

2 tablespoons coconut oil

Honey Butter

½ cup raw honey

⅓ cup coconut oil, almond butter, or sunflower butter

1 tablespoon coconut oil (optional for creamier spread)

1 teaspoon kosher or sea salt

Cornbread makes a great accompaniment to the soups in The Daniel Plan Cookbook as well as a mid-afternoon snack. We recommend having some on hand during the holiday season when comfort foods are in order.

GF DF   6 squares

1. Preheat the oven to 350°.

2. In a medium bowl, fold together flour, flaxseed, baking powder, baking soda, and salt.

3. In another bowl, combine water, honey, applesauce, and oil. Whisk well or use an immersion blender. Pour this mixture over the dry mixture, and whisk together to create a batter.

4. Grease a 7-inch square glass baking dish. Pour in the batter, and spread evenly.

5. Bake for 35 minutes, or until a toothpick inserted into the bread comes out clean. Remove the bread from the oven, and let cool. Cut into 6 even portions.

6. Combine the butter, coconut oil, honey, and salt. This will make a chunky butter to spread over your cornbread.

> **TIP**   Make your own gluten-free cornbread mix by combining 2 cups gluten-free all-purpose flour and 1 cup corn meal.

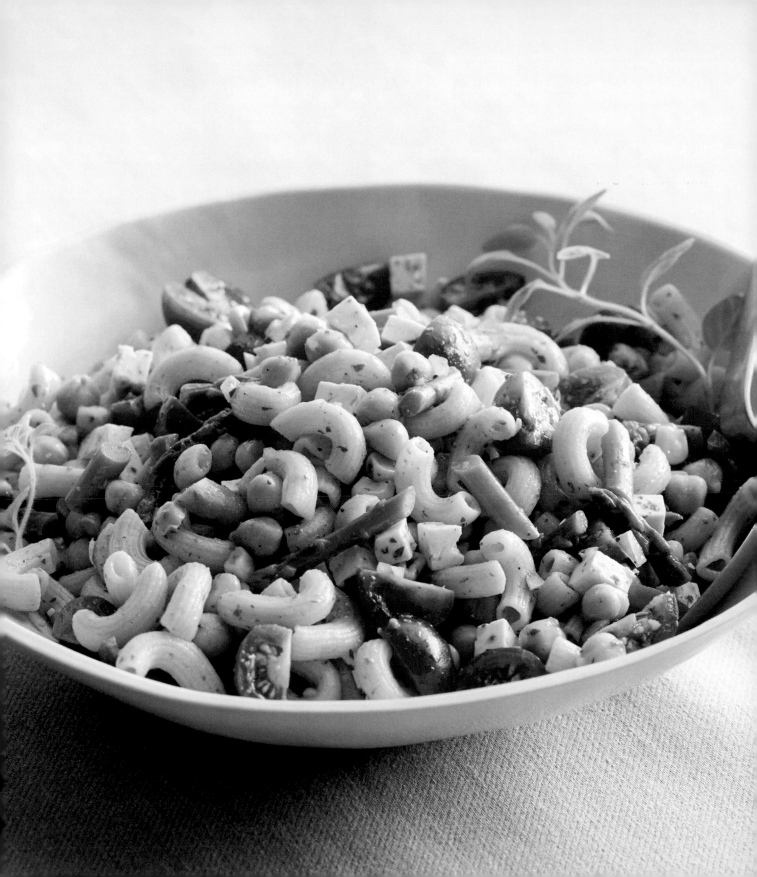

Pasta Salad

8 ounces elbow corn-quinoa pasta

15 spears asparagus, sliced diagonally

18 cherry tomatoes, quartered

4 ounces crumbled feta cheese (omit for DF)

¼ cup finely chopped red onion

¾ cup cooked corn

1 (15-ounce) can garbanzo beans, drained and rinsed

6 tablespoons extra-virgin olive oil, plus extra

¼ cup chopped fresh parsley

¼ cup chopped fresh oregano

3 garlic cloves, minced

2 tablespoons red wine or sherry vinegar

Kosher or sea salt

Black pepper

This pasta salad is easy and colorful. Pack some for a picnic or lunch at work. We've made it gluten-free, but you may use whole wheat or brown rice pasta as well. Choose a small shape such as elbow, penne, or bowtie pasta.

GF **6 servings**

1. Bring a large pot of water to a boil. Cook pasta according to package directions. When pasta is done, remove with a sieve, strainer, or slotted spoon, but keep the water boiling. Drain pasta well, and place in a large bowl. Toss pasta with 1 teaspoon of olive oil to prevent sticking. Allow pasta to cool, stirring occasionally.

2. Drop asparagus into the boiling water, and cook for 2 minutes. Drain and cool.

3. Add the asparagus, tomatoes, cheese, onion, corn, and garbanzo beans to the pasta.

4. Place olive oil, vinegar, parsley, oregano, garlic, salt, and pepper in a blender, and puree. Pour over the pasta and vegetables. Toss gently. Serve chilled or at room temperature.

TIP For a full meal, add grilled shrimp or chicken. Make other variations with zucchini, baby green beans, black olives, other fresh herbs, or chopped arugula or spinach.

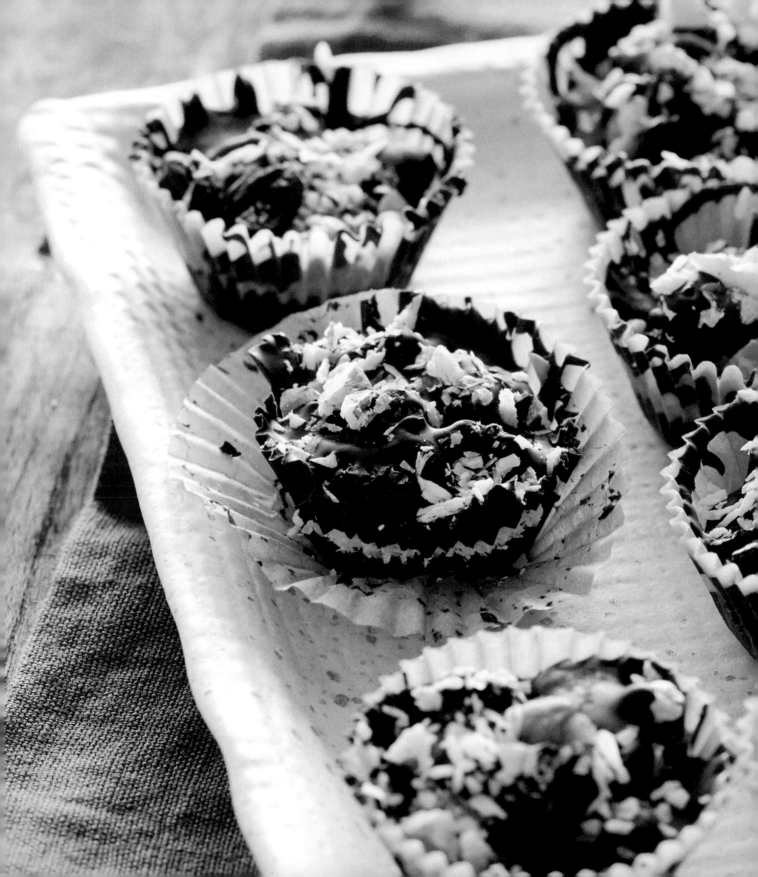

Desserts

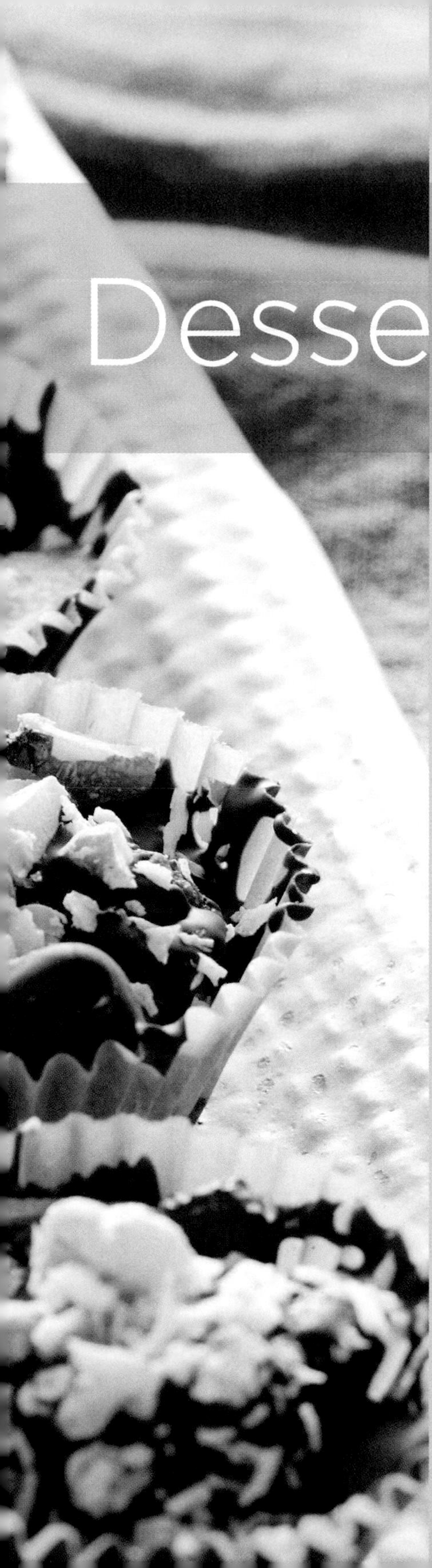

Creamy Gelato

Strawberry Ice Cream

Coconut Hot Chocolate

Chocolate Coconut Pudding

No-Bake Cacao Brownies

◄ Bittersweet Chocolate Cranberry Chews

Baked Oatmeal Chocolate Chip Bars

Ginger Peach Parfait

Cinnamon Maple Apple Crumble

Applesauce Citrus Cake

Creamy Gelato

Raspberry

1 cup coconut water (or regular water)

2 large avocados

⅓ cup raw agave, raw honey, or pure maple syrup

1 teaspoon kosher or sea salt

8 ounces fresh or frozen raspberries

Chocolate (omit raspberries)

1 cup raw cacao

1 teaspoon cinnamon

Orangesicle (omit raspberries)

½ cup orange juice

½ cup diced oranges (or tangerines)

Rich, creamy, and satisfying for any sweet tooth, this gelato also happens to be high in potassium, 100% guilt-free, and good for your brain. Why? This gelato is made from avocados! This recipe is also versatile. Try each variation to find your favorite. **GF** **DF** **4 servings**

1. For basic gelato, place water, avocados, sweetener, and salt into a blender. Blend well, then add in raspberries and puree until rich and creamy. Transfer mixture to an airtight storage container and place in the freezer for 4–6 hours. Serve along with fresh fruit or chocolate sauce.

2. For the chocolate gelato, omit the raspberries, and add the raw cacao and 1 teaspoon of cinnamon to the blender. Freeze 4–6 hours.

3. For the orangesicle, omit the raspberries and blend in the orange juice. After blending, fold in the orange pieces, and then freeze.

THIS GELATO is dairy free, gluten free, free of processed sugars, free of additives, and completely satisfying. It's a great snack to help you avoid a food emergency; eat it any time of the day.

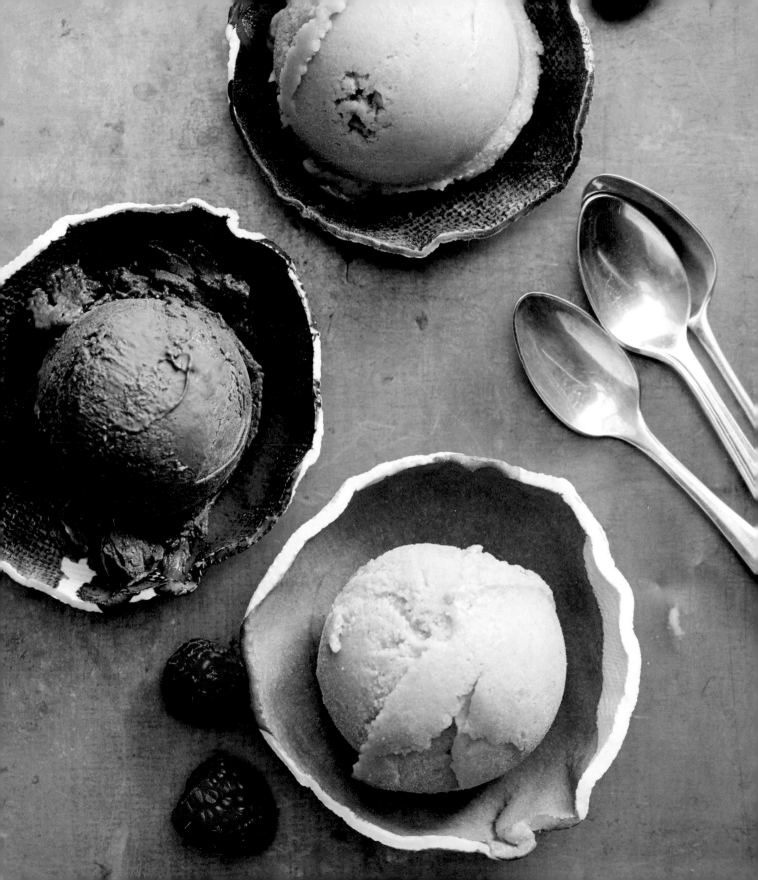

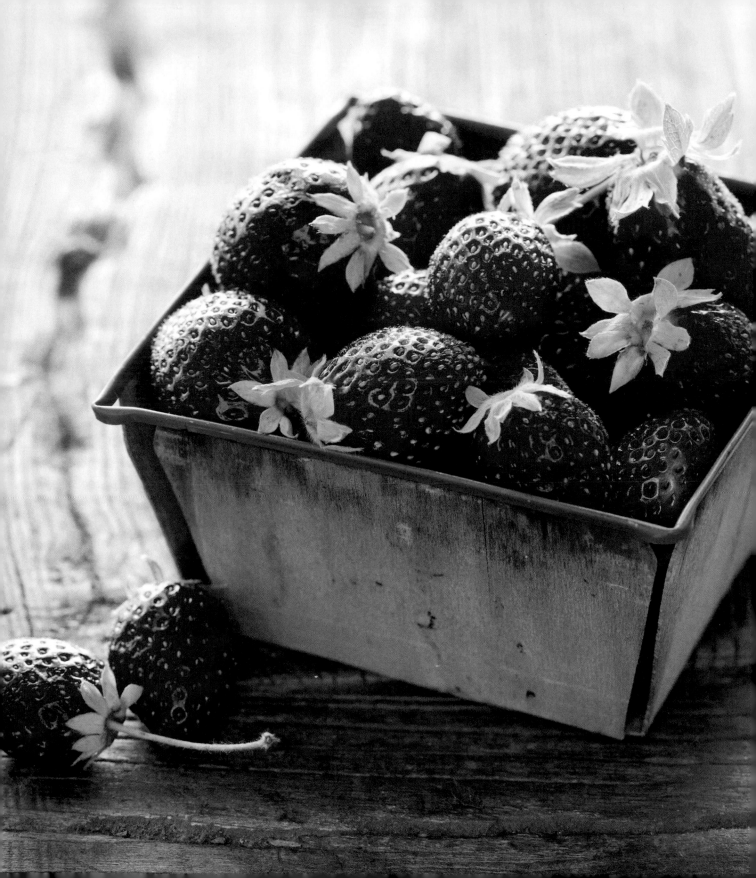

Strawberry Ice Cream

6 ounces unsweetened
coconut milk

2 tablespoons coconut oil

1 teaspoon pure vanilla
extract

12 large frozen
strawberries

Dr. Hyman Favorite

Who says you can't eat ice cream? Typically, ice cream is filled with sugar and heavy cream, but here is a nutritious version that's easy, quick, and tasty! The original version of this ice cream appeared in *The Blood Sugar Solution Cookbook* by Mark Hyman, M.D.

GF **DF** **V**   **3 servings**

1. Chill the freezer bowl of an ice cream maker in the freezer according to manufacturer's instructions before making the ice cream.

2. Combine all of the ingredients in a blender. Blend on high speed until the strawberries are fully broken down and the mixture is creamy, 1–2 minutes.

3. Transfer to the chilled ice cream bowl, and start the machine. When churned, place the ice cream in a sealed container in the freezer until firm, about 3 hours.

Coconut Hot Chocolate

1 (15-ounce) can
coconut milk

1 cup (8 ounces)
almond milk

2 tablespoons Dutch
cocoa powder

2–3 drops liquid stevia
extract

12 ounces 70% bittersweet
chocolate, finely chopped

1 teaspoon pure vanilla or
almond extract

Pastor Warren Family Favorite

Unsweetened cocoa powder is a naturally detoxifying food. Combined with alternative milks, it creates a warm soothing drink.

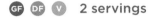 **2 servings**

1. In a small saucepan, bring the coconut and almond milks almost to a boil; turn heat down, and whisk in the cocoa powder, stevia, and chopped chocolate.

2. Stir until smooth, add vanilla, and serve.

> **TIP** Dutch cocoa powder blends more easily with liquid. Increase the cocoa powder to 3 tablespoons for a richer chocolate taste.

Chocolate Coconut Pudding

6 ounces 70% bittersweet chocolate

2 large eggs

10 drops liquid stevia extract (vanilla cream or plain)

1 teaspoon pure vanilla extract

Pinch of kosher or sea salt

1 cup (8 ounces) coconut milk

This rich, smooth pudding takes just a few minutes to make and uses only five ingredients. Use high quality bittersweet chocolate for the best flavor. The portion size is just enough to satisfy a sweet tooth. The recipe doubles easily for a party. **GF DF** **6 servings**

1. Chop chocolate into small pieces. Using a long serrated bread knife or a heavy chef's knife makes it easy. Place chopped chocolate into the bowl of a food processor. Process until very fine. Add the eggs, stevia, vanilla, and salt. Process for a few more seconds.

2. In a small pan over medium heat, bring the coconut milk to a boil. Remove from the heat.

3. Start the food processor, and slowly pour the hot milk through the feed tube. Process until smooth.

4. Divide the hot liquid chocolate equally into six 2-ounce ramekins, dishes, or cups. Refrigerate until chilled and set, about 2 hours.

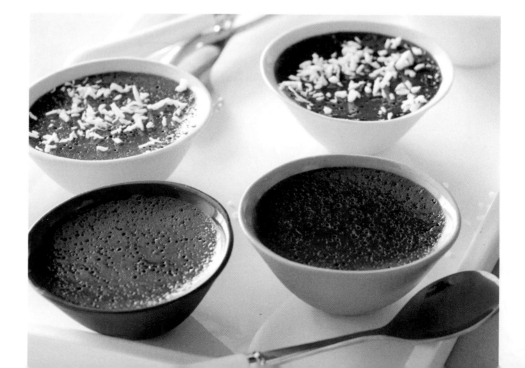

No-Bake Cacao Brownies

4 cups pecan pieces

1 cup raw cacao powder
or Dutch cocoa powder

2 tablespoons cinnamon

1 tablespoon kosher
or sea salt

½ cup raw agave or
raw honey

A quick and easy brownie recipe that is so healthy that you can actually eat it for breakfast (it's deceptively high in protein)! These brownies are delicious topped with the raspberry gelato (page 232) and fresh fruit. Create simple variations by rolling the dough into cookie shapes.

GF **DF** **6–8 brownies**

1. In a food processor, pulse the nuts until they turn into meal. Add the cacao powder, cinnamon, and salt, and pulse again until all materials are combined. Be sure not to overprocess the nuts; otherwise, they will turn into a butter. While pulsing, add the sweetener through the feed tube. A dough ball will naturally form around the blade.

2. Remove the dough, and press the mixture evenly into an 8- or 9-inch square baking pan. Place the brownies in the refrigerator for an hour. Store in an airtight container for up to 2 weeks.

Alternative: If you'd like, spread raspberry gelato over the brownies as a frosting, and freeze for 4 hours. Cut into squares or triangles before serving.

RAW CACAO is different than cocoa powder in that it has not been roasted and contains a higher concentration of minerals. The tasting notes in cacao are similar to coffee beans.

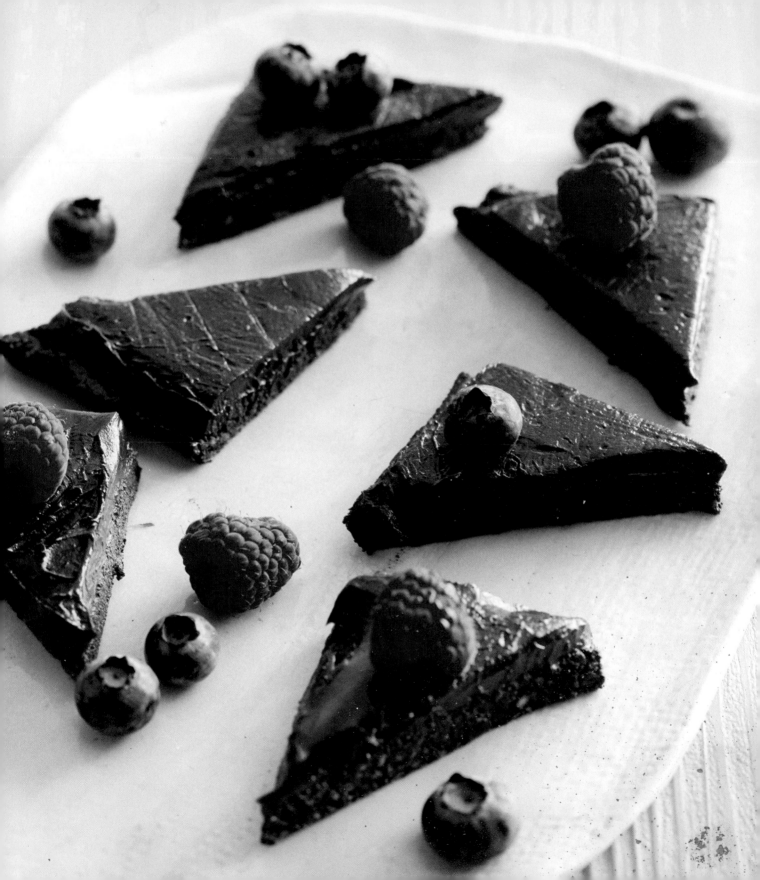

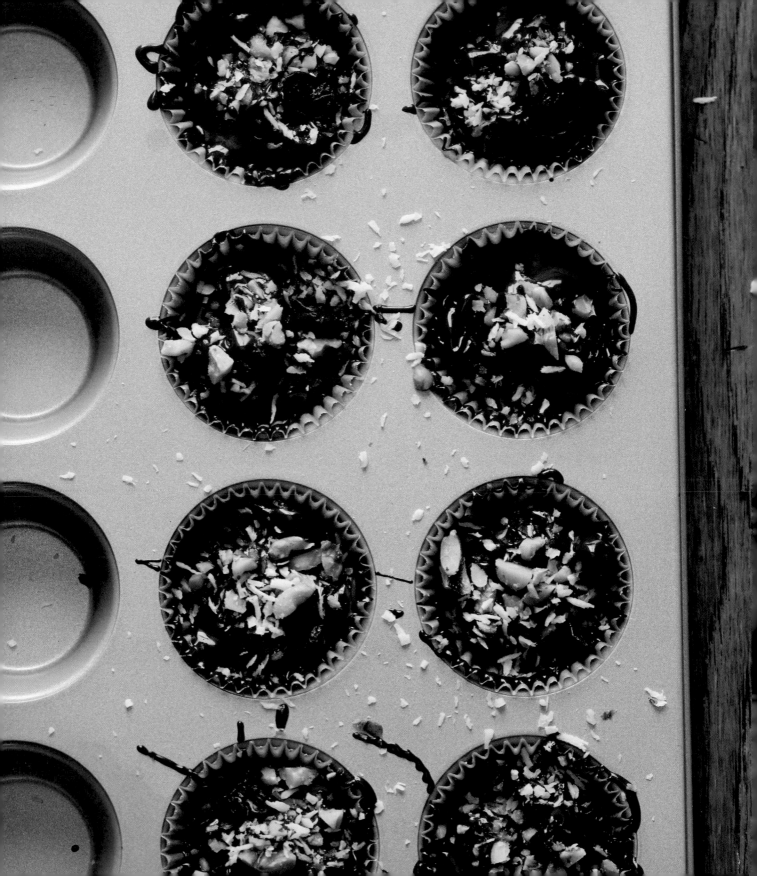

Bittersweet Chocolate Cranberry Chews

4 ounces 70% bittersweet chocolate

¼ cup chopped walnuts

¼ cup dried cranberries

2 tablespoons unsweetened shredded coconut

8 (2-inch) paper baking cups (mini size)

Made with 70% bittersweet chocolate, these delightful little nibbles are portion controlled in mini baking cups. Each bite has about a ½ ounce of chocolate. No cooking required—only melting chocolate. Use high quality chocolate for the best flavor. **GF DF** **8 pieces**

1. With a serrated, bread, or chef's knife, chop the chocolate into small pieces. Melt chocolate either in the microwave or a double boiler.

   To melt chocolate in the microwave: Place chocolate in a microwave-safe bowl. Microwave using 50% power for 1 minute. Remove and stir. Continue in 30-second increments until chocolate is mostly melted. It's ready when there are still a few lumps. They will smooth out as you stir.

   To melt chocolate in a double boiler: Place a few inches of water in a small pan over medium heat and bring to a simmer. Reduce heat to low, and sit a small bowl on top and barely into the pan; it should not touch the hot water. Put chocolate in the bowl. Stir occasionally until chocolate melts smooth.

2. Place 8 paper baking cups on a flat plate, baking sheet, or mini cupcake pan. Drizzle in 1 teaspoon of melted chocolate, then top with a sprinkle of nuts, coconut, and 6–8 dried cranberries. Drizzle with 1 teaspoon melted chocolate, and sprinkle with a bit more nuts and coconut. Refrigerate to set.

Baked Oatmeal
Chocolate Chip Bars

Coconut oil

2 cups old-fashioned
rolled oats

2½ teaspoons cinnamon

1½ teaspoons baking
powder

½ teaspoon kosher
or sea salt

1 cup unsweetened
coconut milk

½ cup unsweetened
applesauce

1 large egg white

4 teaspoons liquid stevia
extract

1¼ teaspoons pure vanilla
extract

1 cup 70% bittersweet
chocolate chunks, finely
chopped

Pastor Warren Family Favorite

When you're craving a chocolate chip cookie, throw together this recipe from Kay Warren for an equally satisfying alternative! Share these tasty bars at a potluck with friends or after dinner with your family. **GF** **DF** **Eight 1-inch bars**

1. Preheat oven to 350°. Brush an 8-inch square pan with coconut oil.

2. Combine oats, cinnamon, baking powder, and salt in a food processor, and pulse to mix well. Or mix well by hand in a large bowl.

3. Add milk, egg white, applesauce, stevia, and vanilla to dry ingredients. Mix well. Gently fold in chocolate chunks.

4. Pour batter into pan. Bake 30 minutes. Remove from oven, and cool slightly before cutting into squares.

TIP Substitute raisins, cranberries, or dried cherries for the chocolate, or reduce the amount of milk and add peanut or almond butter.

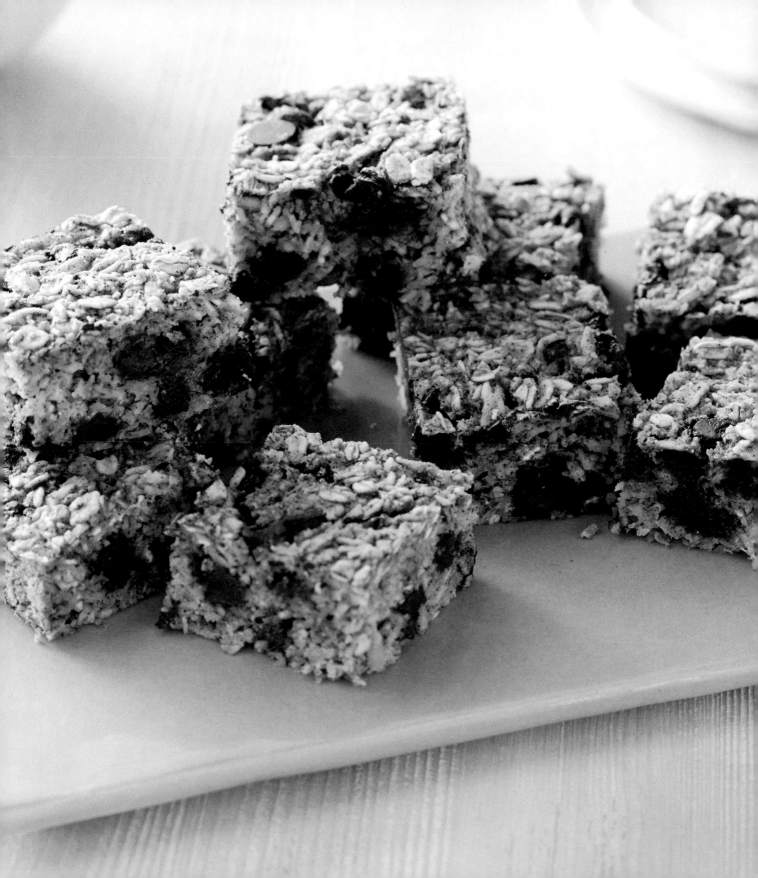

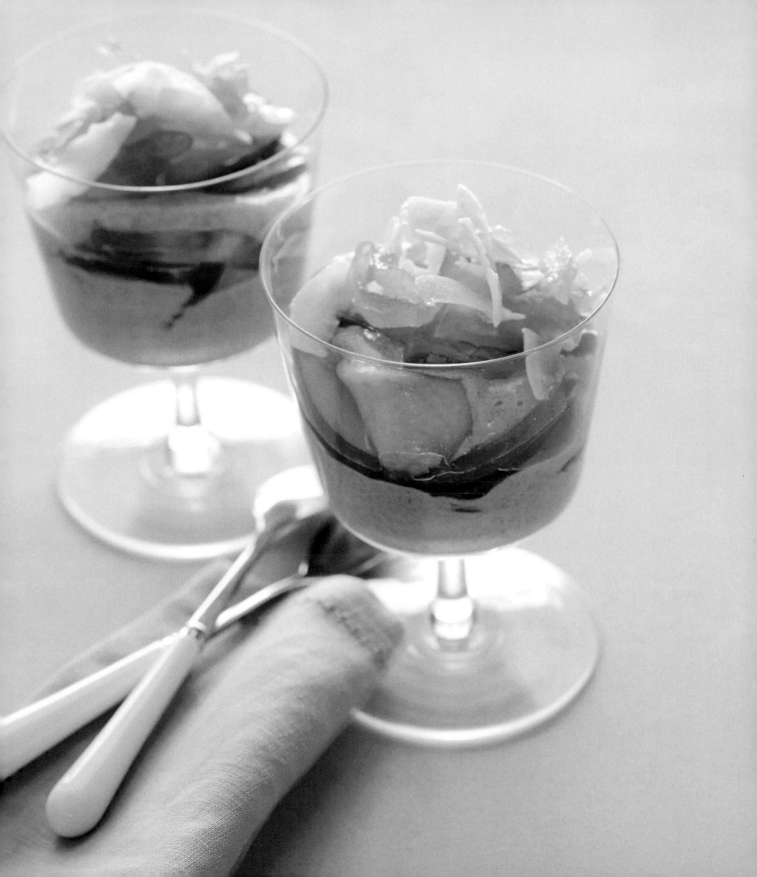

Ginger Peach Parfait

Crème Layer

2 cups macadamia nuts

2 cups water

⅔ cup raw agave or raw honey

2 tablespoons cinnamon

1 tablespoon pure vanilla extract

1 tablespoon kosher or sea salt

Ginger Peach Layer

4 fresh peaches, diced or thinly sliced

2 ounces ginger juice, or 1 tablespoon pumpkin pie spice, or ½ tablespoon dried ginger + ½ tablespoon cinnamon

Topping Layer

⅓ cup dried apricots, thinly sliced

¼ cup shredded coconut

1 tablespoon raw honey

1 teaspoon kosher or sea salt

This parfait can double as a healthy breakfast. It includes three parts that can also be used separately. One trick is to make a little extra of each so you can use the layers for additional toppings and spreads throughout your week. **GF** **DF** **4 servings**

1. Combine crème layer ingredients in a blender. Blend on high until smooth. There should be no pieces of nuts remaining. This layer will save for up to 5 days in the refrigerator.

2. In a medium bowl, toss together the peaches and juice or spices until peaches are coated.

3. In a separate bowl, toss together the topping ingredients.

4. In a fluted glass, layer ¼ cup of the crème layer then ¼ cup of the ginger peach mixture. Repeat, then top with 2 tablespoons of the topping.

Food as Medicine

Macadamia nuts are a rich source of selenium, a heart healthy mineral important to cardiovascular support. Selenium is also essential to healthy blood flow and stimulates the brain to optional functioning. Make your own nut butter by simply processing nuts in a food processor with a pinch of salt (and optional sweetener of choice) until smooth and creamy.

Cinnamon Maple Apple Crumble

Topping

1 tablespoon pure maple syrup

2 teaspoons coconut oil

½ teaspoon pure vanilla extract

¼ teaspoon cinnamon

¼ teaspoon nutmeg

Pinch ground cloves (optional)

½ cup rolled oats

2 tablespoons blanched, slivered almonds

1 tablespoon chopped pecans

2 tablespoons unsweetened coconut flakes or threads

Apples

4 medium apples

4 tablespoons butter (or coconut oil)

4 tablespoons pure maple syrup

½ teaspoon ground cinnamon

Yogurt Sauce

½ cup plain Greek yogurt

2 tablespoons pure maple syrup

Reminiscent of apple pie, these tender apple slices are cooked with a little butter, maple syrup, and cinnamon, then sprinkled with a crunchy topping and a cool yogurt sauce. No refined sugar — just the natural sweetness of maple syrup and apples. What a sweet way to end a dinner!

GF **4 servings**

1. Preheat oven to 300˚.

2. In a small bowl mix together maple syrup, coconut oil, vanilla, and spices until smooth.

3. Add oats, nuts, and coconut, and mix well until evenly coated. Pour onto a rimmed metal baking sheet. Bake for approximately 18 minutes, stirring halfway through. Topping will be fairly dry. Remove from the oven, and allow to cool. Topping will crisp as it cools.

4. Peel and core apples. Cut each apple into 16 pieces.

5. Melt butter and maple syrup together in a medium pan over medium heat. When it is bubbling, add the apple slices and cinnamon. Cook for about 3 minutes, turning and stirring to coat slices. Turn heat to low, and cover with a lid. Cook another 5–7 minutes or until apples are tender when pierced with the tip of a sharp knife. Take the lid off for the last minute or so and allow the apple slices to brown up a bit.

6. Mix yogurt and maple syrup in a small bowl until smooth.

7. Divide apples into bowls, sprinkle with a tablespoon or two of the topping, then a dollop of the maple yogurt. Sprinkle with extra cinnamon if desired.

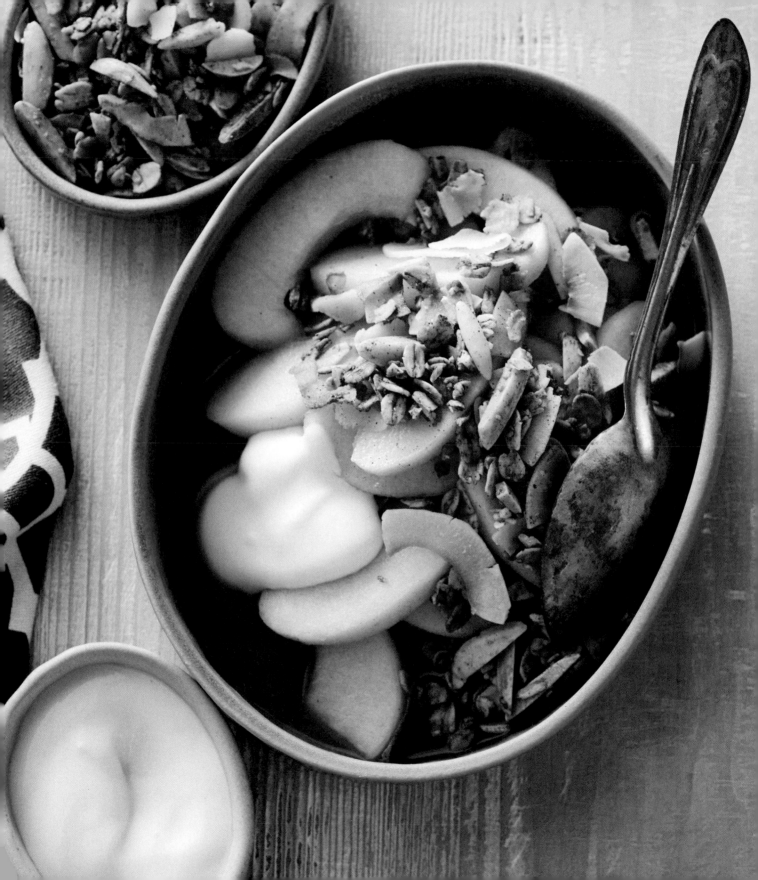

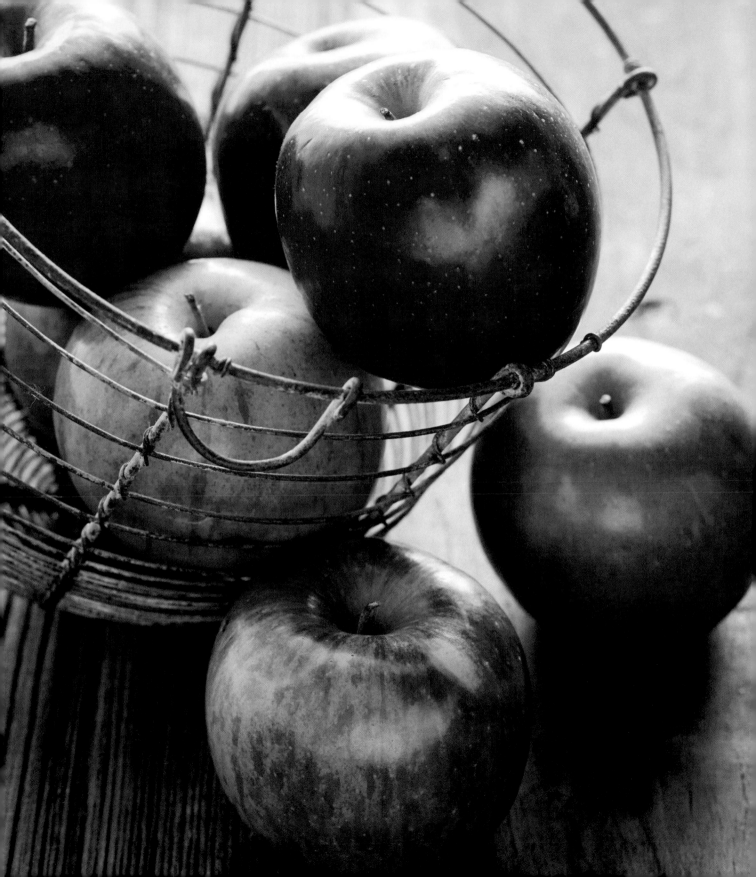

Applesauce Citrus Cake

Coconut oil

2½ cups gluten-free flour

2½ teaspoons baking powder

1½ teaspoons cinnamon

¾ teaspoon baking soda

½ teaspoon nutmeg (or mace)

½ teaspoon kosher or sea salt

2 cups smooth organic applesauce

⅔ cup raw orange blossom or mild honey

½ cup coconut oil, melted if solid

1 egg, beaten

2–3 teaspoons orange zest

1 teaspoon pure vanilla extract

¾ cup chopped walnuts

Moist and sweet from applesauce and spiced with cinnamon and nutmeg, this easy cake makes a satisfying dessert when only something baked will do. It works equally well as a snack cake. It is made with raw honey, instead of refined sugar, and coconut oil proving even dessert can be healthy.

GF DF **10 slices**

1. Preheat oven to 325°. Lightly oil a 9-inch square baking pan, then line with a square of parchment paper cut to fit.

2. In a medium bowl, whisk flour, baking powder, soda, cinnamon, nutmeg, and salt together until well combined.

3. In another large bowl, stir together applesauce, coconut oil, honey, egg, zest, and vanilla until smooth.

4. Pour dry ingredients into the wet ingredients, and stir until completely blended. Stir in walnuts.

5. Pour batter into the pan, and bake until cake is golden brown and a toothpick inserted in the center comes out clean, about 40 minutes. Turn cake out onto a wire rack to cool, remove parchment paper, and slice into 10 pieces. This cake is best enjoyed the day you bake it. However, you may wrap leftovers and store at room temperature for a day or two.

TIP For a creamy sauce to top the cake, use the Greek yogurt sauce from the Cinnamon Maple Apple Crumble recipe (see page 246).

FOR HIGH ALTITUDE ADJUSTMENTS Add 1 tablespoon orange juice, an additional 1 tablespoon flour, and reduce the baking soda and powder by ⅛ teaspoon.

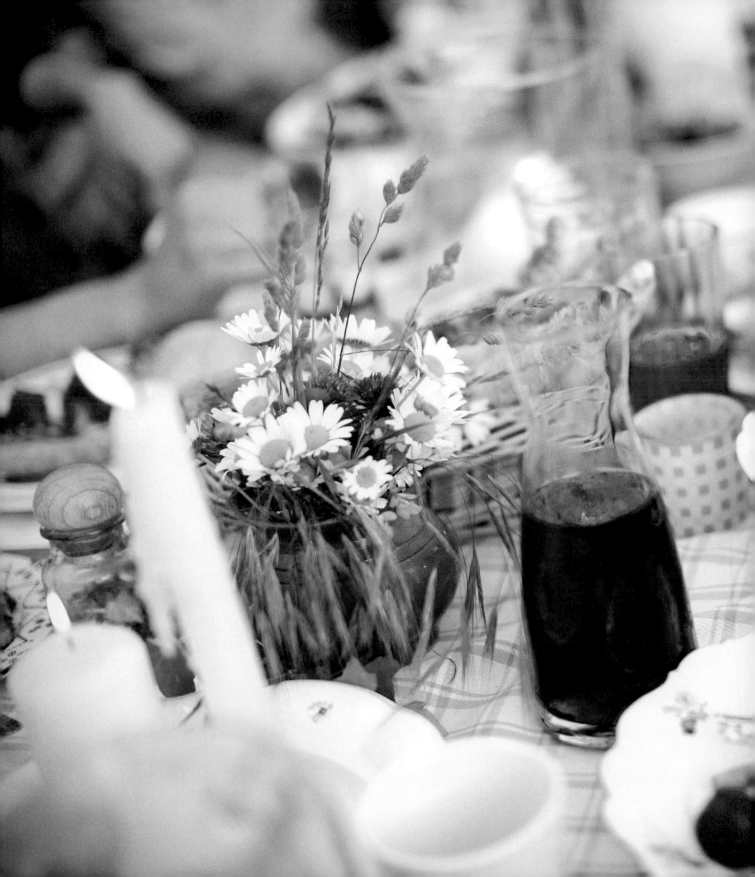

Mealtime Celebrations

What could be more fun than gathering with family and friends to enjoy a meal? Sharing a meal lifts the spirits and fosters a sense of security, well-being, warmth, and love. Eating together facilitates communication and community. When kids are involved, a group or family meal is a great time to model the value of family time, table manners, and healthy eating habits, as well as nurture social skills.

Through The Daniel Plan, we believe we get well in community; it's our "secret sauce." So the most important ingredient in all your recipes are the people you choose to share them with.

We have made getting together for a Daniel Plan–style potluck or party a breeze with fun menus and

(continued)

themes. So go ahead and pick your favorite. Invite your friends and family to join you, and delegate the recipes to guests, or do all the prep work and cooking yourself to serve others. You'll discover the healing power of dining in community.

Party Planning

First, take a head count. How many will be eating? Next, choose a location, such as at your dining table, in your backyard or at a park, or in your church fellowship hall. Enlist volunteers to share responsibilities and make it easy for everyone.

Take a head count to plan for how much food you need.

List all ingredients on a grocery list, multiplying for the number of servings you'll need for snacks, salads, entrees, and desserts.

Plan for extras like beverages, plates, napkins, flatware, or ask guests or family members to bring them.

Shop for all groceries a day or two ahead.

Make appetizers, snacks, or certain elements of your recipes a day ahead of time.

Gather all tools needed to make the recipes, such as baking stones or sheets, salad bowls, serving tools, etc.

Day of the Party

The most important thing is to choose the time you want to eat and work backwards. Allow time for recipes to bake and cool. Get snacks and appetizers out 30 minutes ahead of time. Don't hesitate to ask for help when your guests arrive. Most important, have fun!

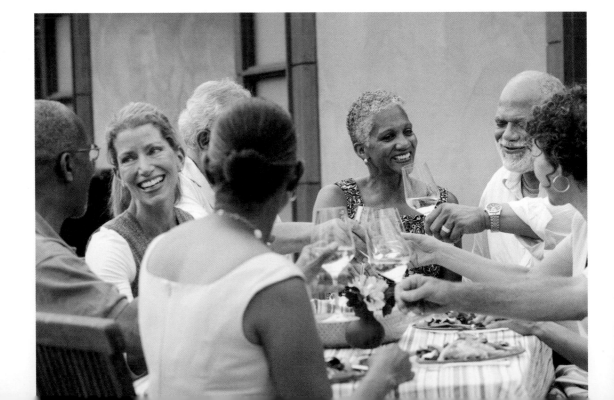

The Daniel Plan Brunch

Brunch offers the best of both worlds: a little sweet and a little savory. This menu combination is great for all ages and allows for a little creative touch of seasonal fruits to be added to dishes.

- Berry Protein Smoothie (page 78) or Very Cherry Smoothie (page 77)
- Gluten-Free Pumpkin Waffles (page 73)
- Garden Patch Omelet (page 67)
- Cobb Salad (page 117) or Shrimp Salad Spring Rolls (page 176)

Day Before: Measure, cut, and slice ingredients for the smoothies, omelets, spring rolls, and salad. Store ingredients separately in the refrigerator. Make the waffles, spring rolls, and separates for the omelet (go ahead and cook them) and salad, and store in the refrigerator.

Day of Party: On the morning of your event, assemble the spring rolls or salad and preheat the oven. Blend the smoothies. Wow your guests right off the bat by filling long fluted glasses with this health-enhancing beverage and putting them on a tray by the door as a welcome snack. Put the waffles in the oven to warm up. Heat a large skillet and cook the omelets according to the number in your party. Plan for ½ an omelet per guest.

For ease of service, plate up a waffle and omelet for each guest then pass the salad and rolls around the table. For refreshing beverages, serve hot or iced cold green tea or even offer a selection of fresh pressed juices.

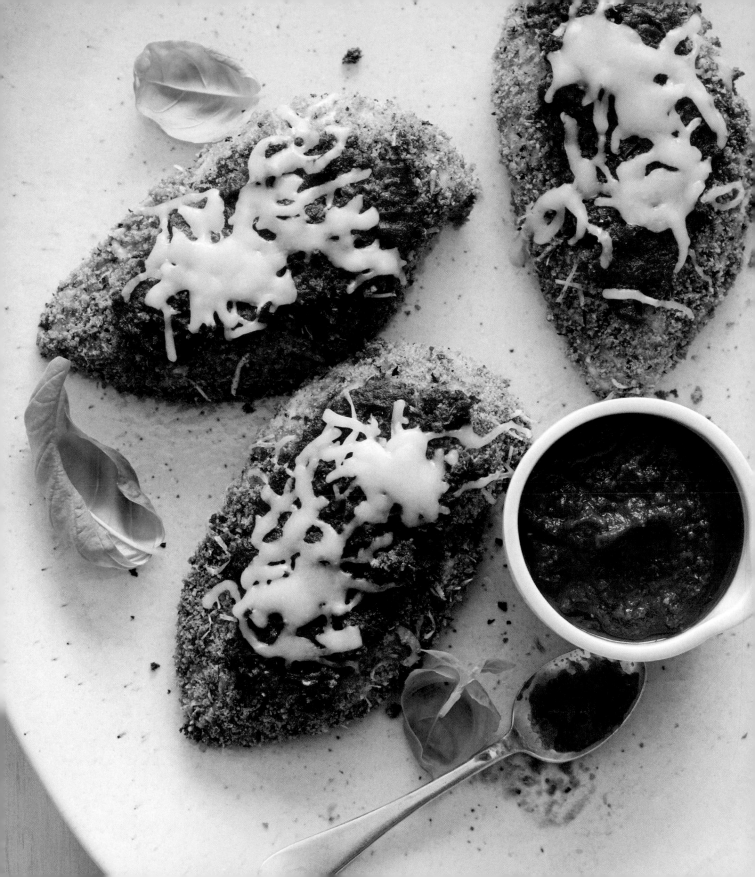

Italian Feast

The celebration and social aspect of food has been a cornerstone of the Italian way for centuries. Take a cue from those food lovers to slow down and enjoy a leisurely feast. This delicious menu offers easy-to-love foods for the whole family as well as recipes that make great leftovers.

- Vegetable Minestrone (page 151)
- Spinach-Stuffed Portabellas (page 175)
- Chicken Parmesan, Pasta Primaverde, or Spaghetti and Meatballs (pages 191, 105, 106)
- Zucchini Pasta (page 113)
- Creamy Gelato (page 232)

Day Before: We recommend making the salad dressing, gelato, and soup, and assembling but not cooking the stuffed mushrooms. Then chop and measure out ingredients for the main entrée. If you decide on spaghetti and meatballs, go ahead and put the ingredients all together, shape the balls, and store in the refrigerator.

Day of Party: One hour prior to guest arrival or the start of your dinner, preheat the oven. Then place the minestrone back in a pot on the stove and heat over low. Remove from heat right before serving. Finish the instructions for the main entrée, then bake the mushrooms, and prep the zucchini noodles and salad. For best results, toss the salad with the dressing, and the pasta and noodles with the sauce immediately before serving. When it's time for dessert, let the gelato sit out for 15 minutes. You might consider scooping the gelato into fun glassware or stemware and serve with toppings like diced strawberries, or dried fruits and nuts.

Fiesta Party

Mexican and Latin cuisine is rich with fresh natural flavors, such as lime, cilantro, and green onions, and broadly appeal to many palates. These perfect Daniel Plan foods — including beans and avocados — are real, whole, and tasty. Most of the Fiesta Party recipes are simple to make and perfect for large groups because many of the recipes can easily be doubled or tripled.

- Spicy Black Bean Soup with Lime and Cilantro (page 147)
- Chips and Guacamole with Fresh Salsa (page 166)
- Avocado Ceviche (page 178)
- Taco Bar (choose your favorites: Grilled Spicy Fish Tacos, Roast Chicken Tacos, Kicking and Screaming Steak Fajitas, or Veggie Tacos) (pages 97 – 102)

Day Before: Any time the day before, prepare the black bean soup, avocado ceviche, baked corn chips, and taco bar ingredients. We even recommend making a little extra of the soup to have for the rest of your week.

Day of Party: Prepare the sauces and guacamole. Grill or cook the meats and veggies for the tacos. Consider cooking a side of brown rice and black beans. Plate all the components into colorful bowls or dishes. Add some fresh cilantro sprigs to the top of the guacamole and fresh fruit to the platter with your dessert.

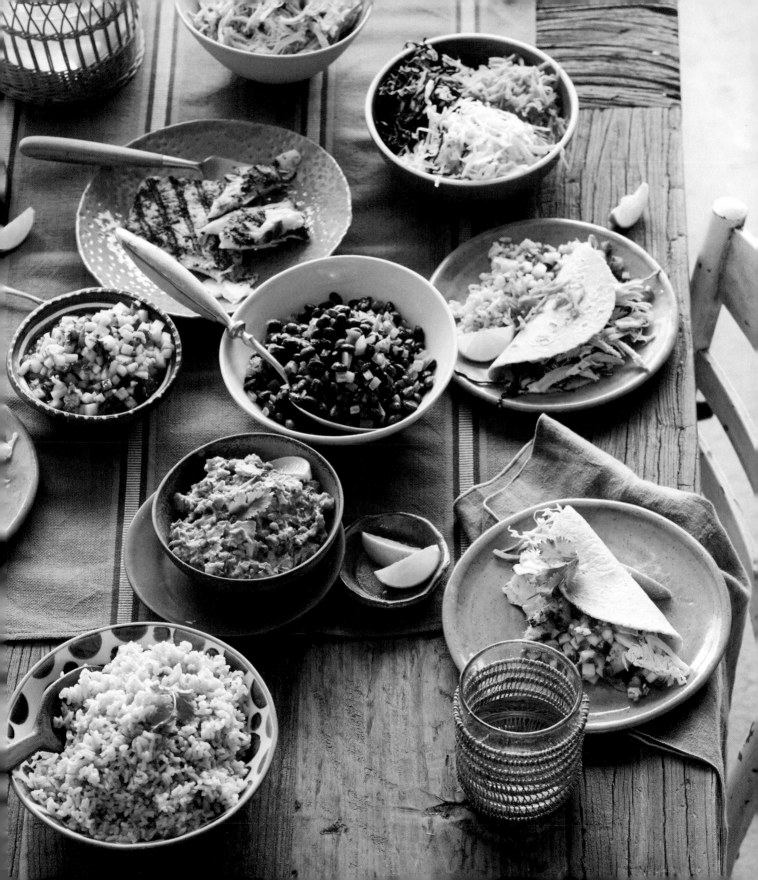

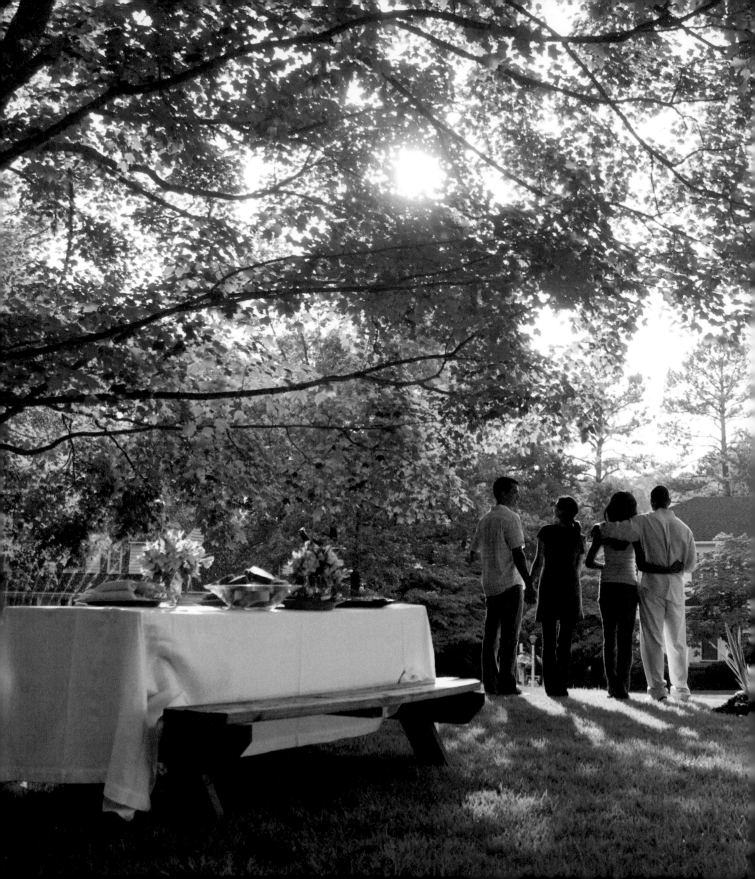

All-American Picnic

Sharing reinvented all-American dishes is ideal for any outdoor gathering. Or take this picnic on the road for a tailgate party or backyard barbecue, or take with you to a church supper.

- Spinach and Artichoke Dip (page 179)
- Burgers: Quinoa-Lentil Veggie Burgers, Herbed Turkey Burgers, or Caramelized Onion Burgers (pages 90 – 94)
- Emerald Broccoli (page 220)
- Sweet Potato Fries (page 225)
- Cinnamon Maple Apple Crumble (page 246)

Day Before: Make the artichoke spinach dip. Cover and let sit in the refrigerator until a half hour before serving time. Bake the chips. Make the pesto and store it in the fridge. Then prep all the parts of your burgers: the patties, the toppings, and the spreads, storing each separately. If you make all three burger recipes, you might elect one condiment and a few vegetable toppings to be used on all three instead of the exact ingredients for each recipe. You could also create smaller patties, cutting the traditional size in half so guests may try each variety.

Day of Party: On the morning of the event, make the apple crumble and bake it. Cool and let sit out on the counter. One hour before your meal, preheat the oven. Make the sweet potato fries, but bake the artichoke dip first then the fries. Heat water for the broccoli and put together the broccoli dish while the fries are cooking.

If you plan to travel with this meal, put each item in its own dish or platter and wrap well with foil (and kitchen towels if you have to drive a ways).

Pizza Party for 12

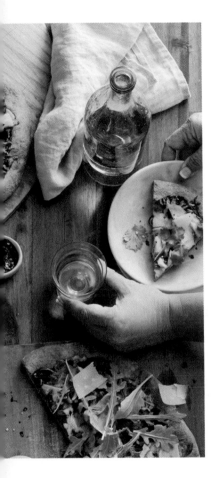

Skip take-out, delivery, or the frozen stuff, and make your own fresh pizza for a pizza party with Daniel Plan recipes.

One 12-inch pizza will serve four people, so figure how many pizzas you will need. Use a single recipe and triple it for three pizzas, or make one of each recipe for a variety of flavors.

Fill in with a big green salad and ice cream for dessert. If you need an appetizer for hungry guests to snack on while the pizzas are baking, put together a platter of raw veggies and two healthy dips.

- Venetian Style Arugula Pizza, Goat Cheese and Turkey Bacon Pizza, and/or BBQ Chicken Pizza (pages 84–87)
- Tangy Caesar Salad (minus chicken) (page 118)
- Hummus (double your favorite Daniel Plan recipe) (pages 170–172)
- Tzatziki Dip (page 173)
- Strawberry Ice Cream (triple batch) (page 235)

Day Before: Make the pizza dough but refrigerate 12–24 hours for a slow rise. Slice and chop vegetables for dips and the salad (use 6 heads of Romaine hearts). Double the salad dressing recipe. Prep all ingredients for the pizza, wrap, and refrigerate separately. Make the ice cream and store in the freezer. Gather all tools such as pizza baking stones or baking sheets, salad bowls, serving tools, and leave out on the counter.

Day of Party: Remove the dough from the refrigerator at least 1 hour before assembling and baking time. Put together salad ingredients but save the dressing until serving time. Set out dips and veggies on your table. Then assemble and bake the pizzas. After the meal, remove the ice cream 20–30 minutes ahead of dessert time to soften.

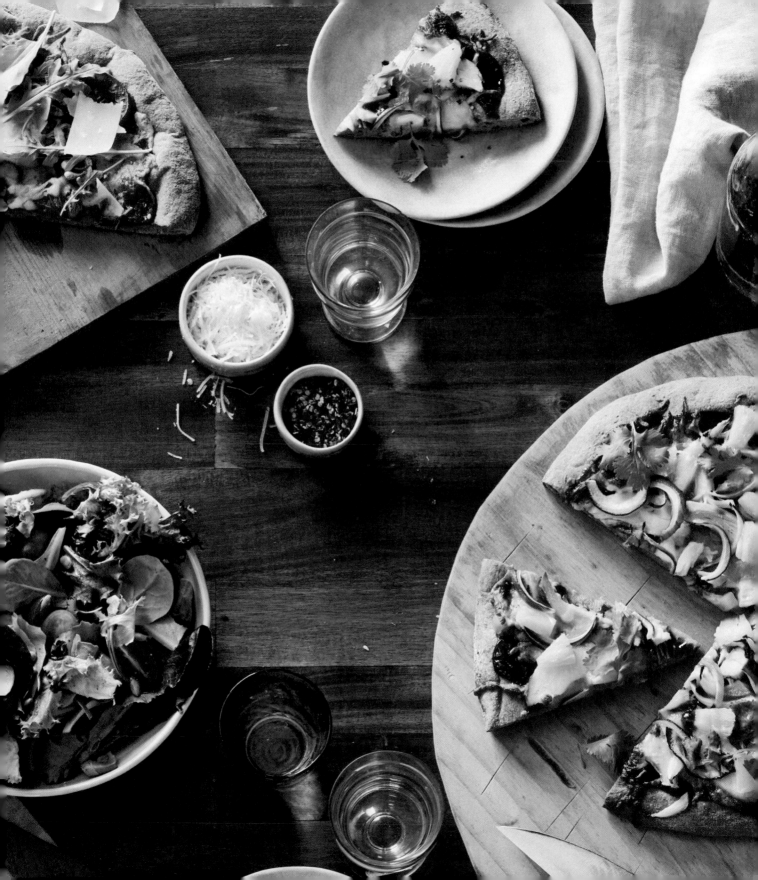

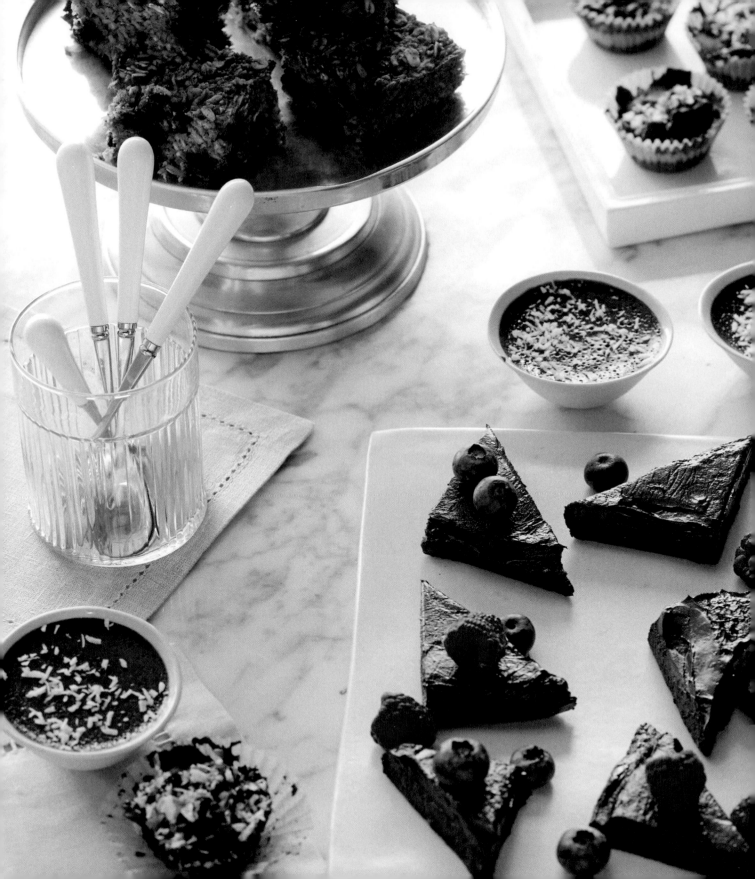

Decadent Dessert Party

Sweet treats are enjoyable on The Daniel Plan because The Daniel Plan dessert tray is truly guilt-free! These desserts can be a joy to share, especially during big celebrations or the holiday season when so many over-the-top desserts show up at parties and dinners.

- Chocolate Coconut Pudding (page 237)
- Applesauce Citrus Cake (page 249)
- Baked Oatmeal Chocolate Chip Bars (page 242)
- Ginger Peach Parfait (page 245)
- No-Bake Cacao Brownies (page 238)
- Bittersweet Chocolate Cranberry Chews (page 241)

Day Before: Prep the parts of the parfait but do not assemble them. Store each item separately. Make the no-bake brownies and chocolate chews (store brownies and chews in the fridge). Measure wet and dry ingredients for the cake and store separately.

Day of Party: On the morning of the event, build the parfaits in parfait or tall glasses and refrigerate them so everything, including the glass, is nice and chilled. Bake the oatmeal bars and let them cool on the counter. Mix the batter for the applesauce cake and bake about an hour and a half before your event. Cut the brownies down into fun shapes using cookie cutters. Display brownies, chews, and oatmeal bars on festive platters or trays. Serve small slices of cake warm and parfaits cold.

This menu would be especially fun served with a variety of hot teas to pair with these delicious desserts.

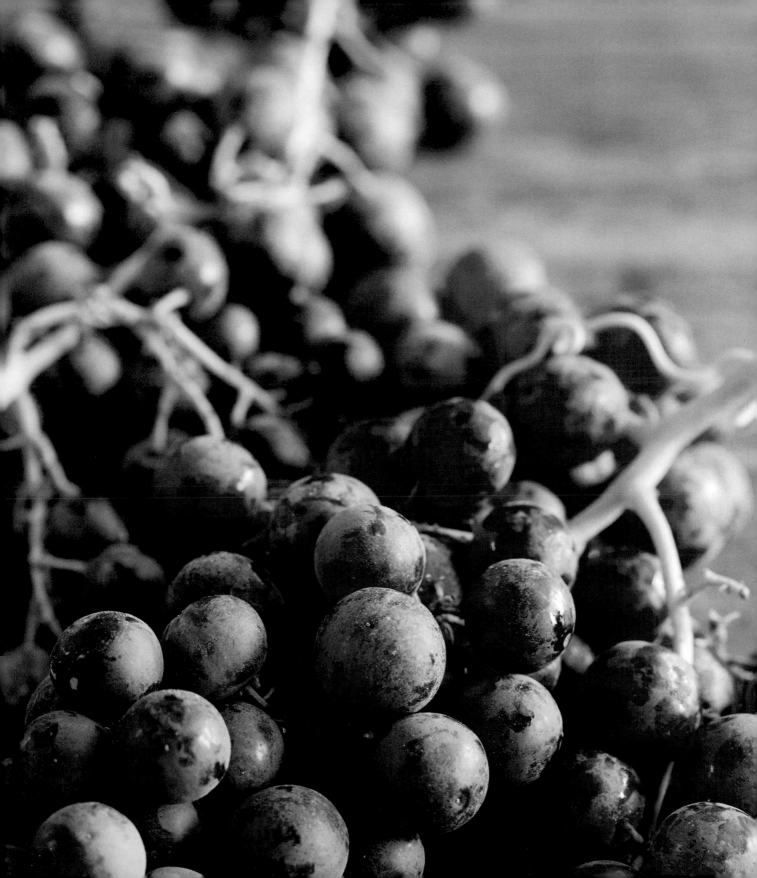

Acknowledgments

With tremendous gratitude, we thank The Daniel Plan chefs — Sally Cameron, Jenny Ross, and Robert Sturm — who understand real food and the value of teaching people to cook and eat healthy. Their time and talents created delicious, easy recipes and so much useful material that will encourage and inspire new and experienced home cooks on their journey toward better health.

From coordinating the recipe testing and revisions to working with the photographers, editors, and designer, Shelly Antol made this cookbook what it is, a user-friendly Daniel Plan guide for the kitchen. Without her project management, this book may never have been born.

Other Daniel Plan team members who contributed their creativity and time: April O'Neil, who wove the value of community into the concept of a Daniel Plan kitchen, and Dee Eastman, director of The Daniel Plan, who provided the overall direction and then trustingly turned it over to the food experts.

This book would not have come to fruition without the beautiful photography and food styling of Matt Armendariz and Adam Pearson and the designs of Ralph Fowler, whose prolific cookbook experience made this book look as appealing to the eye as possible. Andrea Vinley Jewell, our gifted and dedicated editor, gave so much to this project to ensure that high quality marks every page.

From the beginning, Cassie Jones at HarperCollins provided expert guidance on how to create a cookbook that could stand on its own in the marketplace. We are grateful to the entire Zondervan team, specifically to Annette Bourland for seeing the potential and Harmony Harkema for managing the moving parts.

To the many volunteers who tested recipes at home and gave their honest feedback so we could make every single entry enjoyable and tasty, thank you for lending us your kitchens and your taste buds.

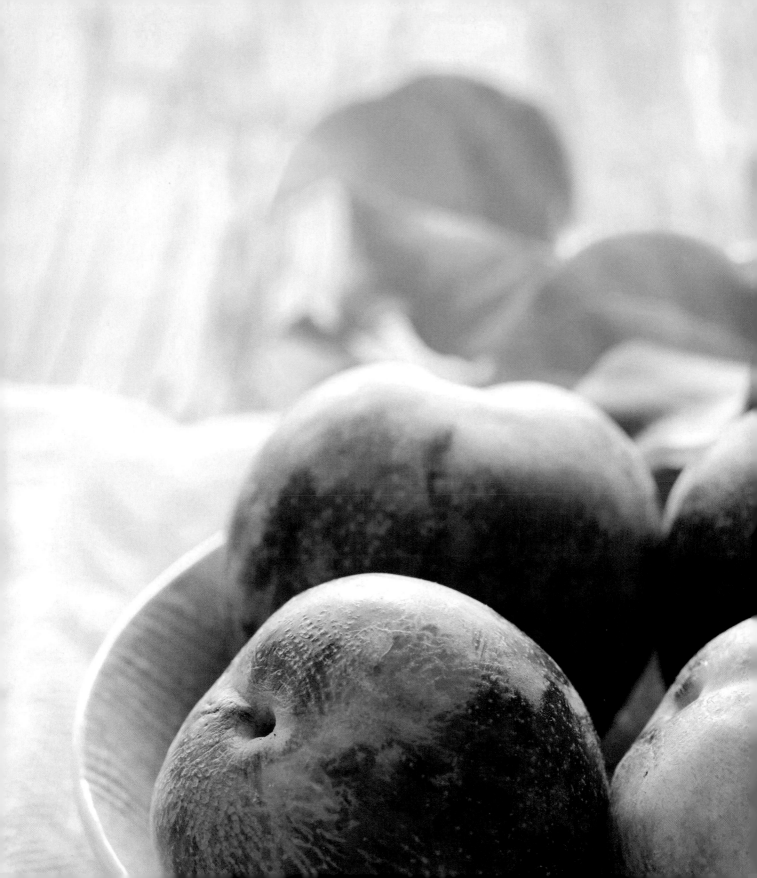

Index

Additional Photo Credits

The Daniel Plan

40 Days to a Healthier Life

Rick Warren D. MIN.
Daniel Amen M.D.
Mark Hyman M.D.

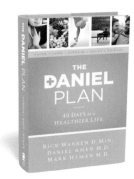

The Daniel Plan: 40 Days to a Healthier Life by Rick Warren, Dr. Daniel Amen, and Dr. Mark Hyman is an innovative approach to achieving a healthy lifestyle where people get better together by optimizing their health in the key areas of faith, food, fitness, focus and friends. Within these five key life areas, readers are offered a multitude of resources and the foundation to get healthy. Ultimately, *The Daniel Plan* is about abundance, not deprivation, and this is why the plan is both transformational and sustainable. *The Daniel Plan* teaches simple ways to incorporate healthy choices into your current lifestyle, while encouraging you to rely on God's power through biblical principles. Readers are encouraged to do The Daniel Plan with another person or a group to accelerate their results and enjoy a built-in support system. Readers are offered cutting-edge, real-world applications that are easy to implement and create tangible results.

Available in stores and online!

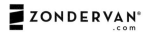

We want to hear from you. Please send your comments about this book to us in care of zreview@zondervan.com. Thank you.

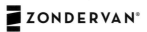